Frontiers In Traumatic Brain Injury

Edited by Xianli Lv, Yi Guo and Gengsheng Mao

Published in London, United Kingdom

Frontiers In Traumatic Brain Injury
http://dx.doi.org/10.5772/intechopen.98165
Edited by Xianli Lv, Yi Guo and Gengsheng Mao

Contributors
Xianli Lv, Huachen Zhang, Hanrui Xu, Shikai Liang, Dominik A. Jakob, Demetrios Demetriades, Jean-Cyrille Pitteloud, Vinu V Gopal, Rinku Raj Mullasseril, Goutam Chandra, Ainat Klein, Wahbi Wahbi, Roy A. Poblete, Grace Y. Kuo, Fawaz Philip Tarzi, Stan Louie, Michael L. Levy, Jillian Plonsker, Michael Brandel, Usman Khan, Youle Su

First published in London, United Kingdom, 2022 by IntechOpen
IntechOpen is the global imprint of INTECHOPEN LIMITED, registered in England and Wales, registration number: 11086078, 5 Princes Gate Court, London, SW7 2QJ, United Kingdom

British Library Cataloguing-in-Publication Data
A catalogue record for this book is available from the British Library

Additional hard and PDF copies can be obtained from orders@intechopen.com

Frontiers In Traumatic Brain Injury
Edited by Xianli Lv, Yi Guo and Gengsheng Mao
p. cm.
Print ISBN 978-1-80356-059-5
Online ISBN 978-1-80356-060-1
eBook (PDF) ISBN 978-1-80356-061-8

Meet the editors

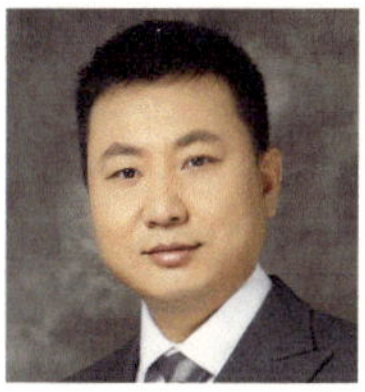

Dr. Xianli Lv, MD, is an Associate Professor of Endovascular Neurosurgery, at the Department of Neurosurgery, Beijing Tsinghua Changgung Hospital, School of Clinical Medicine, Tsinghua University, China. His research focuses on interventional therapy of intracranial aneurysms, cerebral arteriovenous malformation, intracranial dural arteriovenous fistula, spinal vascular malformation, and pediatric cerebrospinal vascular malformations. He is an editorial member of the *Journal of Interventional Neuroradiology, Journal of Stroke and Vascular Neurology, Journal of Neuroradiology*, and *The Neuroradiology Journal*. He is also a deputy editor of *Frontiers in Neurology and Neuroscience Informatics*. Dr. Lv is a member of the World Stroke Organization (WSO) and the World Federation of Interventional Therapeutic Neuroradiology (WFITN) and a consultant for BALT, Montmorency, France.

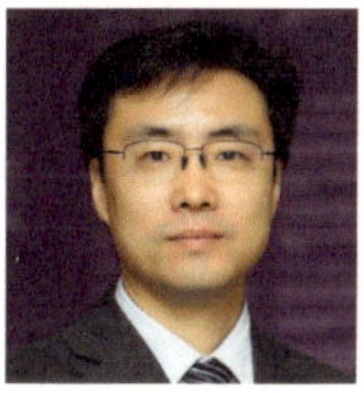

Dr. Yi Guo is an associate professor and deputy director in the Department of Neurosurgery, Beijing Tsinghua Changgung Hospital, School of Clinical Medicine, Tsinghua University, China. His subspeciality is neurovascular surgery and head trauma. In traumatic brain injury research, he focused on the clinical application of cisternostomy and basic research of the glymphatic system. He finished resident training in the Department of Neurosurgery, Affiliated Hospital of Hebei University, and worked there as attending and deputy director. After 2015, he worked in the Department of Neurosurgery, at Beijing Tsinghua Changgung Hospital.

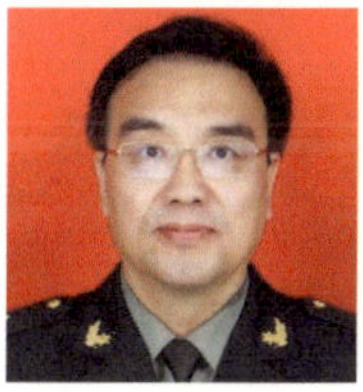

Dr. Gengsheng Mao is a Professor and Director of Neurosurgery, at Chinese PLA General Hospital Third Medical Center. He is the recipient of a Medical Achievement Award from the Chinese Armed Police Forces and a Science and Technology Progress Award from the Chinese Army. He was previously a vice chairman of the Special Committee of Neurorestoratology of the Chinese Medical Association, executive vice chairman and secretary general of the Special Committee of Cerebrovascular Diseases of the Chinese Research Hospital Association, standing committee member of the 10th Army Neurosurgery Special Committee, and vice chairman of the International Society of Neurorestoratology.

Contents

Preface

Traumatic brain injury (TBI) has the highest incidence of all common neurological diseases, making it a huge public health burden. TBI is not only an acute disease but also a chronic disease with long-term consequences, including an increased risk of delayed neurodegeneration. It is a risk factor for a variety of neurological diseases, including epilepsy, stroke, and neurodegenerative diseases and is the leading cause of death among young people as well as the leading cause of death and disability in all ages in all countries. Although research in the field has generated new knowledge about TBI, many needs of TBI patients are not being met. Thus, there is an urgent need to address deficiencies in prevention and care to reduce the huge burden and social costs of TBI. This book discusses the progress of TBI prevention, clinical nursing, research, and challenges in TBI care.

The book is divided into two sections and seven chapters. The first section addresses treatment philosophy. The second section focuses on progress in research and treatment of several complex conditions of brain trauma. Chapter 1 is the introductory chapter, and Chapter 2 discusses prehospital and emergency room airway management in TBI; Chapter 3 examines neuroinflammation in TBI; Chapter 4 reviews penetrating craniocerebral injury in pediatric patients; Chapter 5 discusses traumatic optic neuropathy; Chapter 6 focuses on the traumatic injury of neurovascular arteries and their neurointerventional treatment, and Chapter 7 presents recent advances in the development of biofluid-based prognostic biomarkers of diffuse axonal injury.

We would like to thank all the authors for their contributions. We would also like to acknowledge the encouragement, motivation, and assistance from Tsinghua Precision Medicine Foundation (20219990008), Tsinghua University, China, and the Beijing Municipal Administration of Hospitals Incubating Program (PX2020039. We are grateful to Author Service Manager Blanka Gugic at IntechOpen for her dedication and hard work to ensure the smooth publication of this book. Finally, we owe a debt of gratitude to Professor Zhongcheng Wang, academician of the Chinese Academy of Engineering and the founder and pioneer of Chinese neurosurgery, for without his tireless efforts over the decades, Chinese neurosurgery would not be what it is today.

Xianli Lv
Department of Neurosurgery,
Beijing Tsinghua Changgung Hospital,
School of Clinical Medicine,
Beijing, China

Yi Guo
Beijing Tsinghua Chang Gung Hospital,
Beijing, China

Gengsheng Mao
Chinese PLA General Hospital,
Beijing, China

Dedication

In Memory of Academician Zhongcheng Wang (20th, Dec, 1925-30th, Sep, 2012).

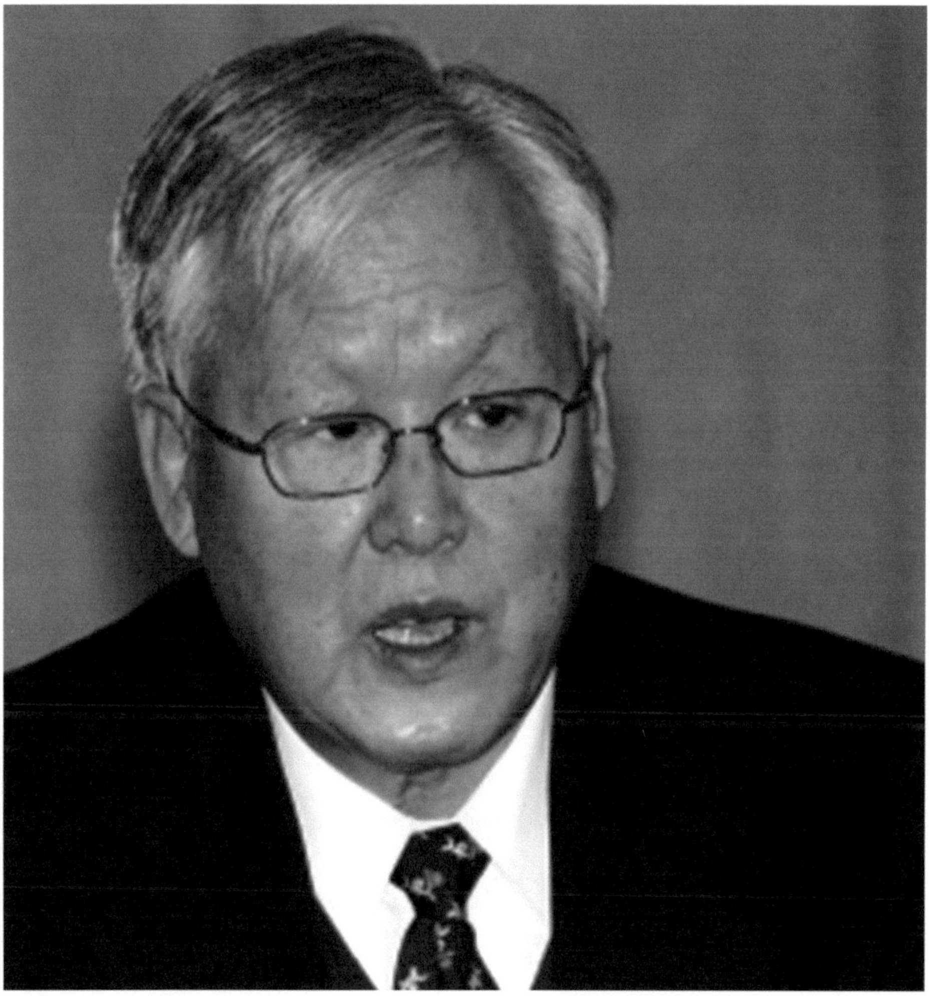

Professor Zhongcheng Wang, academician of the Chinese Academy of Engineering, the founder and pioneer of Chinese neurosurgery, without whose decades' long tireless effort, Chinese Neurosurgery won't be what it is today.

Section 1

General

Chapter 1

Introductory Chapter: Traumatic Brain Injury

Youle Su and Xianli Lv

1. Introduction

Traumatic brain injury (TBI) is a global public health concern and one of the main causes of morbidity, disability, and mortality that has been associated as a risk factor for neurodegeneration and degenerative diseases. Brain injury, secondary to vehicular injury was the most common form of TBI [1]. Yearly, TBI costs the global economy approximately 400 billion US dollars, representing 0.5% of the gross world product [2]. Even with modern diagnosis and treatment, the prognosis for the patient with TBI remains poor. Severe TBI has mortality rates of 30–40% and can cause significant physical, psychosocial, and social deficits in up to 60% of cases [3, 4]. The highest rates of TBI are in children group (0–4 years old) as well as in young age group (15–24 y). There is another high incidence of TBI in old age group (>65 y). The 2 major causes of TBI are falls and motor vehicle accidents generally [5]. Because of the prevalence of TBI, an understanding of the management of this group of patients is vital to the modern health care provider. This introductory chapter based on the 4th edition of the Brain Trauma Foundation guidelines were published in 2016 [6].

2. Pathophysiology of TBI

The pathogenesis of TBI is a complex process, caused by primary and secondary injuries, resulting in temporary or permanent neurological deficits (**Figure 1**) [7]. Primary damage is directly related to the primary external influence on the brain. Secondary injury can occur minutes to days after the primary impact and consists of molecular, chemical, and inflammatory cascades that lead to further brain damage. This cascade involves depolarization of neurons and the release of excitatory neurotransmitters such as glutamate and aspartate, leading to an increase in intracellular calcium. Intracellular calcium activates a series of mechanisms by activating caspases, and free radicals, which lead to cellular degradation, directly or indirectly, through apoptotic processes. This degradation of neuronal cells is associated with an inflammatory response that further damages neuronal cells and triggers disruption of the blood-brain barrier (BBB) and further brain edema. The whole process is also up- and down-regulated through several mediators. The second injury phase is followed by a recovery phase that includes reorganization at the molecular, anatomical, and functional levels.

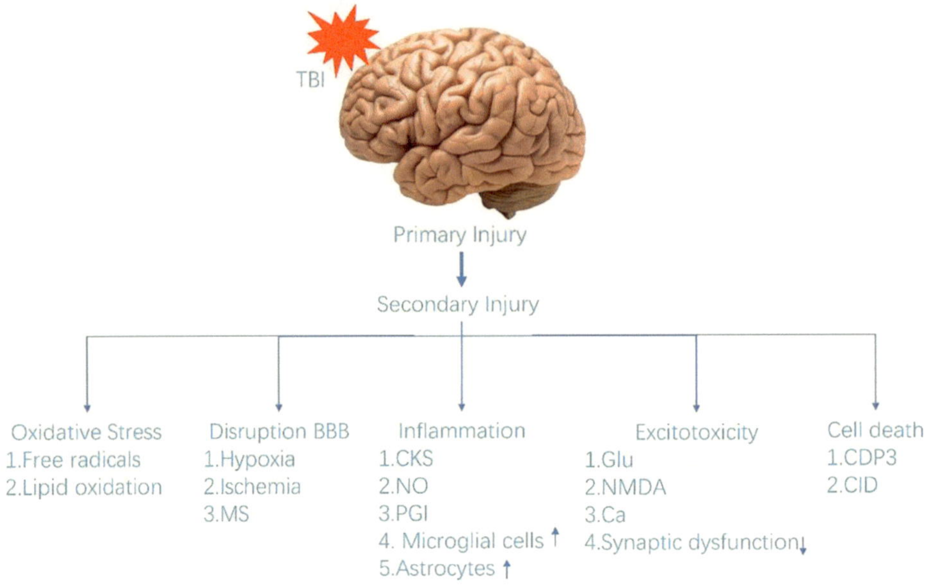

Figure 1.
Secondary injury from oxidative stress, disruption of the blood-brain-barrier (BBB), inflammation, excitotoxicity, and cell death and resulting factors involved in neuronal damage. MS: mitochondrial stress, CKS: cytokines, NO: nitric oxide, PGI: prostaglandins, Glue: glutamate, NMDA: N-methyl-D-aspartate receptor, Ca: calcium, CDP: caspase-dependent 3, CID: caspase-independent factor.

The volume of the intracranial compartment consists of 3 separate contents: brain parenchyma (83%), cerebrospinal fluid (CSF, 11%) and blood (6%). Each of these contents is interdependent on the homeostatic environment within the skull. However, when the intracranial volume exceeds its normal composition, a series of compensatory mechanisms occur. An increase in intracranial volume can occur in the traumatized brain through mass effects of hematoma, cytotoxic and vasogenic edema, and venous congestion. Because brain tissue is incompressible, edematous brain tissue initially causes CSF to squeeze into the spinal compartment. Eventually, blood, especially from venous channels, is also squeezed out of the brain. Without appropriate intervention, sometimes even the maximal intervention, compensatory mechanisms fail, and the end result is pathological brain compression and subsequent death.

3. Neurological exam in TBI

The Glasgow Coma Scale (GCS) is part of clinical practice guidelines and has been commonly used as a bedside neurological scale in routine office practice since its introduction in 1974 [8]. It helps neurosurgeons assess the patient's level of consciousness to determine the severity of TBI in patients. GCS measures eye-opening (4 points), verbal response (5 points), and optimal motor response (6 points), for a total of at least 3 to a maximum of 15 points. This score correlates with changes in pathophysiological changes after TBI and is reflected in the total score; it ranges from 13 to 15 (mild), 9 to 12 (moderate), and less than 8 (severe TBI) [8, 9].

4. Updated medical interventions for TBI

1. Bifrontal decompressive craniectomy is not recommended in severe TBI patients with diffuse injury (no mass lesions) and elevated ICP greater than 20 mmHg for more than 15 min within 1 h, which is not effective for first-line therapy, because it will not improve outcomes as measured by the Glasgow Outcome Score (GOS) at 6 months post-injury [6]. However, this procedure has been shown to reduce ICP and minimize ICU days. Compared with small frontotemporal parietal craniectomy, large frontotemporal parietal decompressive craniectomy (no smaller than 12 cm × 15 cm or 15 cm in diameter) is recommended to reduce mortality and improve neurological outcomes in patients with severe TBI.

2. Although hyperosmolar therapy may lower ICP, there was insufficient evidence about effects on clinical outcomes to support a specific recommendation or to support use of any specific hyperosmolar agent, for patients with severe TBI.

3. Current guidelines do not recommend the use of barbiturates to induce burst suppression measured by EEG to prevent the development of intracranial hypertension. High-dose barbiturates are recommended only to control ICP elevations that are refractory to standard medical and surgical treatment. It is important to maintain hemodynamic stability during barbiturate therapy because patients may develop hypotension.

4. Propofol sedation is recommended for the control of ICP but has failed to show improvement in mortality for 6-month outcomes.

5. The following agents, including Dexmedetomidine and Ketamine, have been shown to have a potential role in the management of TBI patients, although they are not included in the current Brain Trauma Foundation guidelines.

6. Prolonged prophylactic hyperventilation with PaCO2 of ≤ 25 mmHg is not recommended.

7. An EVD (extraventricular drainage) system, which zeroes at the midbrain and continuously drains CSF, can be considered to reduce the ICP burden more effectively than intermittent use. For patients with an initial GCS < 6, CSF drainage may be considered to reduce ICP within 12 h of injury.

8. The use of prophylactic hypothermia, early, within 2.5 h and short-term, 48 h post-injury, is not recommended to improve outcomes in patients with diffuse injury.

9. Once the intracranial hemorrhage has stabilized, low-dose unfractionated heparin or LMWH (low molecular weight heparin) may be used in combination with mechanical prophylaxis. There is a potential risk of intracranial hemorrhage expansion, so the appropriate timing to initiate anticoagulation will be based on clinical guidelines. There is insufficient evidence to support recommendations regarding the preferred drug, dose, or duration of drug prophylaxis for deep vein thrombosis. Other methods, such as compression stockings and maintenance of normovolemia, should be implemented to prevent deep vein thrombosis.

10. When the overall benefits outweigh the complications associated with tracheostomy, tracheostomy is recommended to reduce the number of days on mechanical ventilation to avoid ventilator dysfunction in the patient. Tracheostomy is also considered a potential method to reduce VAP (ventilator-associated pneumonia). However, there is no evidence that early tracheostomy reduces mortality or incidence of hospital-acquired pneumonia. The use of povidone-iodine in oral care to lower VAP is not recommended because it increases the risk of acute respiratory distress syndrome.

11. The use of antimicrobial-impregnated catheters may be considered to prevent catheter-related infections during extraventricular drainage.

12. Feeding patients to attain basal caloric replacement at least by the fifth day and, at most, by the seventh-day post-injury is recommended to decrease mortality. Trans-gastric jejunal feeding is recommended to reduce the incidence of ventilator-associated pneumonia.

13. Prophylactic use of phenytoin or valproate is not recommended for the prevention of advanced PTS (post-traumatic seizures). However, phenytoin is recommended to reduce the incidence of early PTS (within 7 days after injury) because the overall benefit of this treatment is thought to outweigh the complications associated with this treatment. However, early PTS was not associated with worse outcomes. There is insufficient evidence to suggest that levetiracetam is superior to phenytoin in preventing early PTS and toxicity.

14. Steroids are not recommended to improve results or reduce ICP. In patients with severe TBI, high-dose methylprednisolone is associated with increased mortality and is contraindicated.

5. Brain multi-modality monitoring

1. Management of severe TBI patients using information from ICP monitoring is recommended to reduce in-hospital and 2 weeks post-injury mortality.

2. Management of severe TBI patients using guideline-based recommendations for CPP (cerebral perfusion pressure monitoring) monitoring is recommended to decrease 2-week mortality.

3. Jugular bulb monitoring of $AVDO_2$ (Arteriovenous Oxygen Content Difference) may be considered to provide management decisions in TBI patients. Jugular venous saturation < 50% may be a threshold to avoid in order to reduce mortality and improve 3- and 6-month outcomes.

6. Blood pressure thresholds

1. Maintenance of SBP (systolic blood pressure) $\geq$ 100 mmHg for patients 50–69 years of age or $\geq$ 110 mmHg or more for patients aging 15–49 years or 70 years may be considered for reduced mortality and improved outcomes.

2. Recommend treatment for ICP > 22 mmHg, as values above this level are associated with increased mortality.

3. ICP values combined with clinical and brain CT results can be used to make management decisions.

4. The recommended CPP (cerebral perfusion pressure) target for survival and improved outcomes is 60–70 mmHg. Currently, it is unclear whether 60 or 70 mmHg is the minimum optimal CPP threshold and may depend on the patient's autoregulation status.

5. Avoid fluids and vasopressors for CPP > 70 mmHg due to increased risk of respiratory failure.

7. Potential new monitor

The use of brain tissue oxygen tension ($PbtO_2$) monitoring was originally proposed as a method to avoid cerebral ischemia to control ICP during therapeutic hyperventilation. The most common method for monitoring $PbtO_2$ is an invasive probe using a modified Clark electrode, with a typical pathological threshold of 20 mmHg [10]. In multivariate analysis, $PbtO_2$ was shown to have an impact on patient prognosis. This has led to prospective trials of $PbtO_2$-targeted therapy in addition to standard ICP-driven therapy. A phase II trial (BOOST-II, Brain Tissue Oxygen Monitoring, and Management in Severe Traumatic Brain Injury) demonstrated a significant reduction (74%) in the hypoxic burden during hospitalization in the $PbtO_2$-targeted group, with no substantial safety concerns. According to studies, direct intervention is used for ICP management (if >20 mmHg for >5 min), $PbtO_2$ control (if <20 mmHg for >5 min), or both [10]. The third phase of the randomized study (BOOST-III) will evaluate the clinical efficacy of "a treatment regimen based on $PbtO_2$ monitoring compared to a treatment based on ICP monitoring alone" and will enroll patients in the United States.

8. Deep brain stimulation

DBS (Deep Brain Stimulation) has been shown to be effective for cognitive and motor disorders and has the potential to treat other disorders such as depression [11]. These same clinical disorders (e.g., tremor, depression) are frequently present in patients with TBI due to direct structural brain injury or secondary damage from injury. DBS has shown efficacy in the treatment of subgroups of TBI patients with such comorbidities, but the effect of DBS on higher-order function is unclear.

9. Conclusions

TBI is a major global health challenge and priority. Despite the lack of effective treatments for TBI recovery today, continuous efforts have been made over the past few decades to develop therapeutic strategies for TBI recovery. Standard medical and surgical interventions have always played an important role in the acute management of patients with TBI. The number of TBI survivors has increased due to the emergence of better acute management guidelines in the acute phase of TBI, and the number of TBI survivors with various disabilities has increased.

Author details

Youle Su[1] and Xianli Lv[2*]

1 Neurosurgery Department, The Affiliated Hospital of Inner Mongolia Medical University, Huhhot, Inner Mongolia, China

2 Department of Neurosurgery, Beijing Tsinghua Changgung Hospital, School of Clinical Medicine, Tsinghua University, Beijing, China

*Address all correspondence to: lvxianli000@163.com

References

[1] Maas AIR, Menon DK, Adelson PD, Andelic N, Bell MJ, Belli A, et al. Traumatic brain injury: Integrated approaches to improve prevention, clinical care, and research. Lancet Neurology. 2017;**16**(12):987-1048

[2] Taylor CA, Bell JM, Breiding MJ, Xu L. Traumatic brain injury-related emergency department visits, hospitalizations, and deaths—United States, 2007 and 2013. MMWR Surveillance Summaries. 2017;**66**(9):1-16

[3] Marehbian J, Muehlschlegel S, Edlow BL, Hinson HE, Hwang DY. Medical management of the severe traumatic brain injury patient. Neurocritical Care. 2017;**27**(3):430-446

[4] Vella MA, Crandall ML, Patel MB. Acute management of traumatic brain injury. The Surgical Clinics of North America. 2017;**97**(5):1015-1030

[5] Galgano M, Toshkezi G, Qiu X, Russell T, Chin L, Zhao LR. Traumatic brain injury: Current treatment strategies and future endeavors. Cell Transplantation. 2017;**26**(7):1118-1130

[6] Farrell D, Bendo AA. Perioperative management of severe traumatic brain injury: What is new? Current Anesthesiology Reports. 2018;**8**(3):279-289

[7] Crupi R, Cordaro M, Cuzzocrea S, Impellizzeri D. Management of traumatic brain injury: From present to future. Antioxidants (Basel). 2020;**9**(4):297

[8] Mena JH, Sanchez AI, Rubiano AM, Peitzman AB, Sperry JL, Gutierrez MI, et al. Effect of the modified Glasgow Coma Scale score criteria for mild traumatic brain injury on mortality prediction: Comparing classic and modified Glasgow Coma Scale score model scores of 13. The Journal of Trauma. 2011;**71**(5):1185-1193

[9] Dikmen SS, Machamer JE, Powell JM, Temkin NR. Outcome 3-5 years after moderate to severe traumatic brain injury. Archives of Physical Medicine and Rehabilitation. 2003;**84**(10):1449-1457

[10] Khellaf A, Khan DZ, Helmy A. Recent advances in traumatic brain injury. Journal of Neurology. 2019;**266**:2878-2889. DOI: 10.1007/s00415-019-09541-4

[11] Kundu B, Brock AA, Englot DJ, Butson CR, Rolston JD. Deep brain stimulation for the treatment of disorders of consciousness and cognition in traumatic brain injury patients: A review. Neurosurgical Focus. 2018;**45**(2):E14

Chapter 2

Prehospital and Emergency Room Airway Management in Traumatic Brain Injury

Dominik A. Jakob, Jean-Cyrille Pitteloud and Demetrios Demetriades

Abstract

Airway management in trauma is critical and may impact patient outcomes. Particularly in traumatic brain injury (TBI), depressed level of consciousness may be associated with compromised protective airway reflexes or apnea, which can increase the risk of aspiration or result in hypoxemia and worsen the secondary brain damage. Therefore, patients with TBI and Glasgow Coma Scale (GCS) ≤ 8 have been traditionally managed by prehospital or emergency room (ER) endotracheal intubation. However, recent evidence challenged this practice and even suggested that routine intubation may be harmful. This chapter will address the indications and optimal method of securing the airway, prehospital and in the ER, in patients with traumatic brain injury.

Keywords: prehospital, emergency room, endotracheal intubation, airway, outcomes, traumatic brain injury

1. Introduction

Traumatic brain injury (TBI) is frequently associated with depressed level of consciousness, compromised protective airway reflexes or apnea, which can increase the risk of aspiration or result in hypoxemia and worsen the secondary brain damage. Therefore, patients with TBI and Glasgow Coma Scale (GCS) ≤ 8 have been traditionally managed by prehospital or emergency room (ER) intubation. This practice is also reflected by the current guidelines: the American College of Surgeons Committee on Trauma Advanced Trauma Life Support (ATLS) recommends intubation for patients with a GCS of 8 or lower for airway protection [1]. Also, the practice management guidelines of the Eastern Association for the Surgery of Trauma give a level 1 recommendation for endotracheal intubation of patients with severe cognitive impairment (GCS ≤ 8) [2].

However, the potential benefit of an intubation in TBI, is also associated with risks: Difficult or failed endotracheal intubation may cause hypoxemia, aspiration, and hypotension and requires admission to the intensive care unit (ICU). In fact, there is no direct evidence supporting routine intubation of all patients with a GCS ≤ 8. Consequently, recent evidence challenged the practice of a strict GCS threshold for intubation and even suggested that routine endotracheal intubation for GCS ≤ 8 in TBI may be harmful [3].

The primary goal in the prehospital care of the trauma patient is to secure adequate ventilation until transfer to hospital care. To achieve this goal, various techniques for airway establishment and subsequent ventilation can be performed: endotracheal intubation has been considered as the gold standard. However, ventilation may also be achieved by less invasive and time consuming procedures such bag-valve mask (BVM) ventilation with the optional use of oropharyngeal (OPA) or nasopharyngeal (NPA) adjuncts. More advanced techniques include supraglottic airway (SGA) devices. There is a wide range of medications available to facilitate intubation prehospital or in the ER.

To date, there are no evidence-based guidelines for TBI patients regarding standardized airway management in the prehospital setting or in the ER. This explains also why indications and techniques for airway establishment vary in different systems and countries around the world. In the United States of America (USA) prehospital care is usually provided by emergency medical technicians or trained paramedics, whereas prehospital care in most European countries is provided by physicians [4]. Following these differences of American and European Emergency Medical Service (EMS) systems, the US prehospital care strategy follows more "scoop and run approach" with prioritizing rapid patient transport to trauma centers. In Europe the priority lies more on field triage, on scene assessment and initiation of procedures such as intubation "stay and play approach" [5].

This chapter will address the question what airway management strategy best meet the patients need and is associated with most favorable outcomes in TBI. Indications and optimal method of securing the airway prehospital and in the ER will be discussed. In addition, technical aspects including medication for pretreatment, induction, paralysis and sedation for endotracheal Intubation in the presence of TBI will be outlined.

2. Prehospital airway management

Advanced prehospital care has been practiced for several decades in Western countries. In TBI particularly, prehospital airway management is one of the most critical aspects that determine patient outcomes. The importance of the airway management is reflected by the Advanced Trauma Life Support (ATLS) algorithm [1], in which the airway takes priority over any other therapeutic interventions.

General prehospital TBI guidelines [6] are emphasizing avoidance and treatment of hypoxia, prevention and correction of hyperventilation, and avoidance and treatment of hypotension. The implementation of these prehospital guidelines showed that adjusted survival doubled among patients with severe TBI and tripled in the severe, intubated cohort. Furthermore, guideline implementation was significantly associated with survival to hospital admission [7]. These findings support the widespread implementation of the prehospital TBI treatment guidelines. However, specific evidence-based guidelines are needed to establish the optimal airway management in the prehospital setting.

Patients require an advanced airway under two sets of circumstances: failure to maintain a patent airway and the inability to oxygenate and ventilate the patient adequately [8]. While endotracheal intubation in the OR is a very safe and straightforward procedure with very low complication rate, emergency intubation of an unstable patient in the field is linked to a high rate of complication with up to 25% mortality in some studies. Emergency intubation remains a hazardous maneuver even under the best conditions. And no matter how skilled the prehospital team is, best conditions are seldom encountered in the field. This is why endotracheal intubation should ideally performed by skilled providers in patients who are likely to benefit from this technique. In a prehospital setting the indication to establish an airway is not always that obvious and depends on multiple factors (**Figure 1**) [9].

a. Severity of patients' condition and the presence of hypoxia: Traumatic brain injury (TBI) is frequently associated with depressed level of consciousness, compromised protective airway reflexes or apnea, which can increase the risk of aspiration or result in hypoxemia and worsen the secondary brain damage. During the past 45 years, the quantitative GCS as a simple and practical numeric method for assessing impairment of the level of conscious has become the universal criterion for mental status assessment [10]. Consequently, the GCS is also a frequently used score to decide whether an intubation should be performed or not. According to the ATLS [1] and the practice management guidelines of the Eastern Association for the Surgery of Trauma [2] intubation is recommended for GCS ≤8. However, there is no scientific evidence supporting this practice. The dogma that patients with a GCS ≤ 8 are at higher risk for aspiration or hypoxic injury has now been challenged. A prospective study from Hong Kong, in 2012, showed that of 33 patients with a GCS ≤ 8 36.4% had intact airway reflexes and potentially

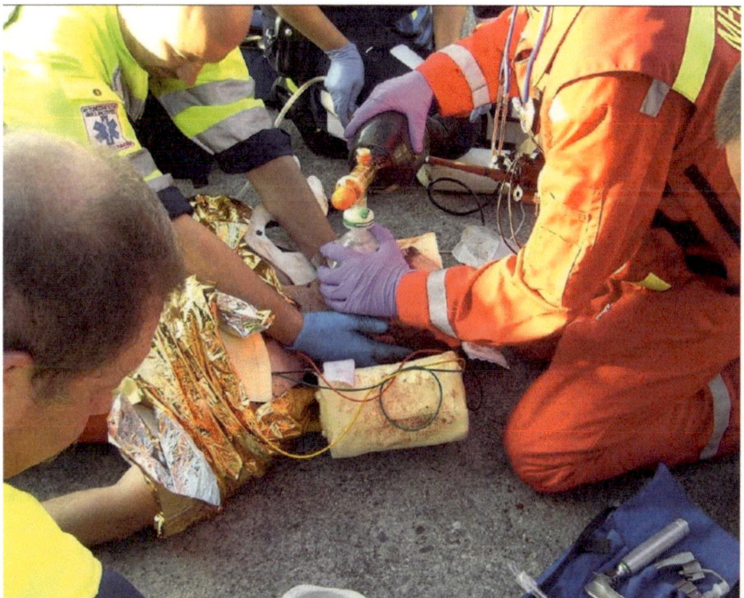

Figure 1.
Prehospital airway-management. The indication to establish an airway in a prehospital setting depends on: the severity of patients' condition and the presence of hypoxia; the training and skills of the EMS personnel including the available equipment; and the safety and environment on scene. Figure provided by Clerc EMS Monthey, Switzerland.

capable of maintaining their own airway, whilst many patients with a GCS > 8 have impaired airway reflexes and potentially be at risk for aspiration [11].

The need for immediate establishment of an obstructed or impaired airway or hypoxia is unquestionably associated with better outcomes. However, performing an intubation in a suboptimal environment in the field, especially if performed by paramedics, may be challenging and require multiple attempts and in some cases may result in the loss of airway with catastrophic consequences. A difficult intubation may result in hypoxemia, aspiration, and hypotension, factors that may contribute to worse outcomes. Also, prehospital intubation and hand ventilation is often associated with hyperventilation and hypocapnia, which could worsen brain edema and secondary brain damage. Finally, prolonging the prehospital time and delaying definitive care, may have adverse effects on the patient, especially in the presence imminent herniation due to increased intracranial pressure (ICP) or an ongoing hemorrhage.
In conclusion, it is important to identify those patients who might benefit from prehospital endotracheal intubation and those who can potentially be harmed by the procedure. At this moment there is no class I evidence supporting any specific approach. It might be appropriate to attempt prehospital intubation in a small number of selected patients with imminent airway obstruction or hypoxia not responding to oxygen administration.

b. Training and skills of the EMS personnel and the available equipment: In the United States of America (USA) prehospital care is usually provided by emergency medical technicians for basic life support (BLS) or trained paramedics for advanced life support (ALS), whereas prehospital care in most European countries is provide by physicians. Basic providers are restricted to splinting, bandaging, alignment of displaced limbs, the administration of oxygen including BVM ventilation, chest compression and the use of an automated external defibrillator (AED) in case of cardiac arrest. However, especially in the USA many of BLS providers have obtained an intermediate level (EMT-I); these individuals can obtain a more definitive airway such as using a SGA device or even perform endotracheal intubation. Paramedics are trained and performed endotracheal intubation. However, very often many paramedics, especially in areas with no large trauma volumes may not use this skill very often and may become less competent with the procedure. On the other hand, especially an experienced physician proficient with endotracheal intubation, is more likely to perform an intubation more liberally, often unnecessarily. In the United States, prehospital care strategy follows the principle of "scoop and run" with prioritizing rapid patient transport to trauma centers and minimal interventions on scene. In Europe there is a strong element on field triage and initiation of more advanced therapeutic interventions, such as intubation. This prehospital strategy is also known as "stay and play". A matched cohort study compared patients with isolated severe TBI in Switzerland and the United States [12]. In line with the described differences in prehospital strategies, patients in Switzerland had significantly longer scene times (23 vs. 9 minutes, $p < 0.001$) and prehospital endotracheal intubation was more frequently performed (31% vs. 18.7%, $p = 0.034$). However, no significant differences in outcomes were observed between the two cohorts. The results what prehospital strategy should be prioritized and if an endotracheal intubation should be performed remain controversial, although there is evidence that a "scoop and run" approach is preferable for penetrating trauma. In these scenarios the number of meaningful interventions that can be made by prehospital providers is limited and rapid transportation to the hospital is the most important aspect, because in-hospital surgery is typically needed for hemorrhage control.

c. Safety and environment on scene: The safety aspect on scene, as well as the transportation mode and the expected time to reach the next hospital are important for considering airway interventions on scene. Especially for longer transports, the time-saving aspect of the scoop and run approach without airway interventions becomes less important and early establishment of an airway may improve patient outcomes.

Considering all factors above, complexity of the decision to perform a prehospital intubation becomes obvious, and it is not surprising that the literature on this topic remains contradictory. A retrospective multicenter study including 13,625 patients with moderate to severe TBI showed that prehospital intubation was independently associated with a decrease in survival [13]. Several other studies implicated out-of-hospital intubation as a factor associated with negative outcomes [14, 15]. In a recently published study prehospital airway management in severe TBI patients did not have a significant impact on mortality or long-term neurological outcomes [16]. Other investigations have also demonstrated no difference or even improved outcomes with field intubation [17, 18].

Besides intubation, different other options for airway management are available in a prehospital setting. The simplest approaches such as the jaw thrust or chin lift maneuver are included in the first aid. Oropharyngeal (OPA) or nasopharyngeal (NPA) adjuncts may be inserted orally or nasally to secure an open airway. More advanced airway techniques include the establishment of an airway using an SGA device and finally the performance of endotracheal intubation. In particular cases, a surgical airway must also be considered. A major challenge in prehospital airway management is to determine the appropriate approach for the individual patient in the present environment and setting. **Table 1** shows various airway management techniques and summarizes advantages and disadvantages in prehospital use.

A recently published systematic review [19] was assessing comparative benefits and harms across three different airway management approaches (BVM, SGA, and endotracheal intubation) for patients with trauma, cardiac arrest, or medical emergencies requiring prehospital ventilatory support or airway protection. Overall, 99 studies involving 630,397 patients from 1990 to September 2020 were considered for analysis. The evaluated outcomes included mortality, neurological function, return of spontaneous circulation (ROSC), and successful advanced airway insertion. Different meta-analyses were stratified first by study design (RCTs or observational studies), and then by emergency type (cardiac arrest, trauma, medical) and population age (adult, pediatric, mixed-age). All meta-analyses outcomes were reported as favoring one of the two compared approaches, or no difference. Sufficient evidence was not available to address all outcomes and all patient characteristics, provider characteristics, and variations in techniques that were specified a priori. For adult trauma patients 1-month post incidence survival was not different when BVM was compared to endotracheal intubation. Other comparisons for adult trauma patients did not show sufficient evidence to favor an airway management strategy over another. Potential harms of airway management for the entire study population were also compared. When comparing BVM vs. SGA and BVM vs. endotracheal intubation, no difference

Airway management techniques	Skills	Training needed	Time needed	Possible complications	Level of sedation/ unconsciousness needed	Equipment needed	Protection against aspiration and airway shutdown	Ventilation possible without face mask
Manual	Trauma jaw thrust, trauma chin lift	+	+	–	+	–	–	–
Simple	Oropharyngeal airway, Nasopharyngeal airway	++	++	+	++	+	–	–
Advanced	Laryngeal mask, laryngeal tube	+++	++	+	++	++	(+)	++
Definitive airway	Endotracheal intubation, surgical airway	++++	++++	++++	++++	++++	++++	+++

Table 1.
Overview of different airway management techniques—advantages and disadvantages in prehospital use.

was found. When comparing SGA to endotracheal intubation, SGA was superior in terms of multiple insertion attempts; endotracheal intubation was superior in terms of inadequate ventilation. No difference was recorded for aspiration, oral/airway trauma and regurgitation. The authors concluded that the currently available evidence does not indicate benefits of more invasive airway approaches based on survival, neurological function, ROSC, or successful airway insertion. However, most included studies were observational. This supports the need for high-quality randomized controlled trials to advance clinical practice and EMS education and policy, and improve patient-centered outcomes.

3. Airway management in the ER

Similar to the prehospital setting the standard indications for an advanced airway establishment in the ER, include low GCS, failure to maintain a patent airway and the inability to oxygenate and ventilate the patient adequately. In the presence of a TBI a diminished level of consciousness with the concern for the loss of airway control is very common and likely the most frequent indication for ER intubation. Therefore, the GCS is most commonly used to decide whether an intubation should be performed or not.

Patients with TBI and a GCS ≤ 8 have been traditionally managed by ER endotracheal intubation. However, this practice is based mainly on expert opinion and long-standing dogma. There is very little evidence to support this policy! Recent work has challenged this practice! A recently published study including patients with isolated severe head injuries suggested that routine endotracheal intubation in the ER for GCS of 7 and 8 may be even harmful [3]. In this study 2727 patients with GCS 7/8 and isolated blunt head trauma were included. Overall, 1866 (68.4%) patients were intubated within 1 hour of admission (immediate intubation), 223 (8.2%) had an intubation >1 hour of admission (delayed intubation), and 638 (23.4%) patients were not intubated at all. After correcting for age, gender, overall comorbidities, tachycardia, GCS, alcohol, illegal drug use, and head injury severity, immediate intubation was independently associated with higher mortality (OR 1.79, CI 95% 1.31–2.44, $p < 0.001$) and more overall complications (OR 2.46, CI 95% 1.62–3.73, $p < 0.001$).

A study [20] evaluating a general trauma population with GCS of 6–8 came to a similar conclusion. An intubation within 1 hour of arrival was associated with an increase in mortality and longer ICU and overall length of stay compared to patients without an intubation. The authors also performed a subgroup analysis of patients with head injury and found similar results to that of the overall trauma population.

These two studies showing worse outcomes associated with immediate intubation and suggest that the existing GCS threshold to mandate intubation in patients with isolated head injuries should be revisited.

Beside the GCS, additional clinical criteria may help to guide the decision to intubate TBI patients in the future. A recently published study showed that head abbreviated injury scale (AIS), tachycardia and younger age were independent clinical factors associated with intubation [3]. These factors could potentially be taken into account to formulate a more selective approach to immediate intubation. In the mentioned study a policy of intubating all isolated blunt head injury patients ≤ 45 years with head AIS 5 and GCS 7 would have improved intubation management, with 7 immediate instead of delayed intubations and only three potentially unnecessary intubations. If these defined criteria are met (high specificity), an early intubation should be strongly considered. On the other hand, the defined criteria are not suitable to identify patients who definitely do not require an intubation (low sensitivity). Future research should focus on defining more adequate clinical parameters to identify patients requiring immediate intubation and should avoid fixed GCS threshold.

Muakkassa et al. [21] compared trauma patients who were intubated because of combativeness, and not because of medical necessity. In line with the findings above intubating for combativeness was associated with longer hospital LOS, increased rates of pneumonia, and worse discharge status when compared with matched non-intubated patients. It appears that the risks and adverse events of intubation may outweigh the potential benefits of intubation in specific trauma populations.

Therefore, the following potential risks associated with intubation in TBI patients need to be considered by every health care provider. Laryngoscopy and the endotracheal tube can cause a sympathetic or parasympathetic stimulation. Sympathetic stimulation may increase heart rate, blood pressure [22] and ICP [23], whereas parasympathetic stimulation can trigger bronchospasm or hypotension. Especially the increase in ICP from the sympathetic surge can cause an increase in cerebral blood volume, cerebral edema, and development of worsening hemorrhage or hematoma. Finally, both, sympathetic and parasympathetic stimulations may increase mortality and brain injury.

Ventilation after intubation need to be monitored closely, because both hyper- and hypoventilation can contribute to worse outcomes. Severe hyperventilation (arterial pCO_2 below 25 mm Hg) should be avoided due to the risk of vasoconstriction and cerebral ischemia. In general, a normo-ventilation with an arterial pCO_2 within 35–45 mm Hg should be targeted. However, mild hyperventilation (arterial pCO_2 within 30–34 mm Hg) is commonly used to address high intracranial pressure and may potentially be beneficial [24]. More important to address the elevated ICP in TBI patients is the initiation of hyperosmolar therapy with mannitol or hypertonic saline when additional bleeding is suspected [25].

Technical aspects and medications for endotracheal intubation carries also risks for TBI patients. The following section gives an overview including recommendations for pretreatment, induction, paralysis, and sedation of patients with TBI to prevent secondary brain damage.

4. Technical aspects including medication for pretreatment, induction, paralysis and sedation for endotracheal intubation in the presence of TBI

Endotracheal intubation remains the gold standard for airway management in trauma patients and should be performed via the oral route and a manual in-line stabilization maneuver [26]. Rapid sequence induction (RSI) is widely used for emergency intubation and often considered as the gold standard for trauma patients. This technique uses a fast acting anesthetic in combination with a fast acting relaxant to achieve rapid intubation. Only a few people are aware that this technique was formally described by P. Safar back in 1970 [27]. The primary goal of this technique was to prevent regurgitation during induction of anesthesia in patients with bowel obstruction. Hypoxemia and hypotension were hardly considered at that time, when advanced monitoring and pulse oximetry were still tools of the future. From today's point of view, this technique is not ideally suited to prevent hypoxemia and hypotension. While in standard OR practice, such short events will hardly result in more than a check on the Q/A sheet, they may have devastating consequences on outcomes in patients with TBI.

In addition, complication rate increases significantly with the number of intubation attempts, with a sharp increase if more than 2 attempts are needed [28]. This suggests that first pass success should be the gold standard in emergency intubation, and return to basic maneuvers or surgical airway should be considered if 2 attempts have failed.

Another important aspect is efficient airway clearance before intubation, which has been shown to significantly increase first pass success [29]. That is why suction of the airway, while having little relevance in the OR can be a game changer in emergency intubation.

Good oxygenation throughout the procedure is paramount in brain injured patients, so meticulous attention should be paid to optimizing precondition. A recent study [30] has shown that when intubation is attempted in a patient with a $SpO_2 < 93\%$, there is almost 100% incidence of severe hypoxemia while incidence goes down to 17% if SpO_2 is 95% or more. While optimizing oxygenation status may take some time, it certainly pays off in terms of patient outcome.

Last but not least a close monitoring during intubation is mandatory. Studies have shown that episodes of hypoxemia during intubation attempts often go unrecognized, both in the field and in the ER. Furthermore, after intubation attention should be taken to avoid hyperventilation as it can cause hypocapnia and thus cerebral vasoconstriction; it also can impair venous return leading to hypotension. As trivial as it might seem, having a team member watching the vital signs is an important factor in the intubation process.

In the following section medication for pretreatment, induction, paralysis and sedation for endotracheal intubation in the presence of TBI are discussed.

There is currently no evidence to support the use of intravenous lidocaine as an intubation pretreatment for RSI in patients with TBI [23]. High-dose fentanyl (at 2–3 mcg/kg) can help to blunt the sympathetic stimulation of intubation and is currently recommended for neuroprotection in patients with increased ICP.

In TBI the induction with etomidate is popular all over the world because of its mild hemodynamic profile. Particularly, in TBI a drop in mean arterial pressure (MAP) and the subsequent decrease in cerebral perfusion pressure (CPP) may have devasting consequences. It's important to be aware that etomidate has no analgesic properties, and neuroexcitation may need to be addressed separately.

Ketamine for induction is a good option, with the additional benefit of analgesic properties. The concern of sympathetic stimulation, leading to an increase in ICP is no longer valid. On the contrary, ketamine may, in fact, be neuroprotective due to an increase in MAP and CPP [31], without an increase in cerebral oxygen consumption or reducing regional glucose metabolism [32]. Ketamine may best be used for induction in the presence of hypotension because of for the described effect of increasing MAP and CPP [33].

For paralysis succinylcholine or rocuronium can be utilized [34]. Succinylcholine, as a depolarizing neuromuscular blocking agent has the advantage of rapid onset and offset properties, which is beneficial in TBI patients regarding early neurological examinations. Rocuronium on the other hand can lead to delays in proper neurological examinations due to prolonged paralysis. A retrospective study of 2016 compared 233 TBI patients requiring intubation in the ER. RSI was either performed with succinylcholine or rocuronium. Overall mortality rate was similar between the two groups. However, for patients with a high head AIS score (4–6), succinylcholine was associated with increased mortality compared with rocuronium (44% vs. 23%, odds ratio (OR) 4.10, 95% confidence interval (CI) 1.18–14.12; p = 0.026). Prospective studies are need to clarify these findings.

Propofol in TBI patients for post-intubation sedation is widely used and has the advantage of rapid onset of action and short duration of action. However, since it has no analgesic effect, it needs to be combined with medication for pain control. Furthermore, care should be taken in hypotensive patients because it may lower the MAP and subsequently the CPP. For post-intubation continuous sedation, a combination of propofol and fentanyl in the normotensive or hypertensive patient is therefore recommended. Fentanyl is a potent analgesia without appropriate sedation properties. While the hemodynamic properties of fentanyl are relatively stable, a decrease in MAP and HR frequently occur due to the cessation of the sympathetic stimulus triggered by pain. In addition, an increase in ICP has been described in several studies. A minimal appropriate dose for TBI patients is therefore recommended.

In hypotensive patients a combination of midazolam and fentanyl or ketamine alone is a good option. Midazolam as a sedative has the additional benefit of anxiolytic and anticonvulsant properties. Compared to propofol the effect on ICP and CPP are comparable. However, it's important to have in mind that the onset and offset action of midazolam is initially relatively fast but tissue accumulation over time may be associated with delayed awakening. This is particularly disadvantageous in patients with TBI, as rapid clinical assessment after cessation of the drug is wanted.

A relatively new approach for emergency intubation is the delayed sequence induction (DSI) technique described by Weingart and colleagues [35]. In contrast to RSI, the technique of delayed sequence intubation temporally separates administration of the induction agent from the administration of the muscle relaxant to allow adequate pre-intubation preparation. This technique uses ketamine sedation to optimize preoxygenation with CPAP or assisted ventilation before muscle relaxant is given and intubation performed. Recent studies have shown an improved safety profile in emergency intubation using this technique. A ketamine-only breathing intubation, in which ketamine is used without a paralytic is another promising alternative. In this case the patient continues to breathe spontaneously, while ketamine provide hemodynamic benefits compared to standard RSI and is also a valuable agent for post-intubation analgesia and sedation. When RSI is not an optimal airway management strategy, ketamine's unique pharmacology can be harnessed to facilitate alternative approaches that may increase patient safety [36].

5. Conclusion

Airway control is particularly important for patients with TBI because hypoxemia and hypercarbia may cause secondary brain damage.

In a prehospital setting the indication to establish an airway depends on multiple factors such as (a) severity of patients' condition including the presence of hypoxia, (b) the training and skills of the EMS personnel including the available equipment, (c) the safety and environment on scene.

In the presence of a TBI a diminished level of consciousness with the concern for the loss of airway control is very common and likely the most frequent indication for intubation. Traditionally patients with TBI and Glasgow Coma Scale (GCS) ≤ 8 have been managed by prehospital or ER endotracheal intubation. However, recent evidence challenged this practice and even suggested that routine intubation may be harmful. There is evidence that intubation according to a strict GCS threshold is associated with risks and adverse events that may outweigh the potential benefits of intubation in TBI patients. Future research should focus on defining more adequate clinical parameters to identify patients requiring immediate intubation and should avoid fixed GCS threshold. Furthermore, less invasive airway management strategies such as BVM ventilation or the use of SGA devices may be equally effective and potentially associated with less complications. The cornerstone of prehospital airway management should focus on aggressive prevention and treatment of hypoxemia, hypotension, and, if the patient receiving positive pressure ventilation, prevention of hyperventilation. If an intubation is performed in a TBI patient induction with etomidate or ketamine in the presence of hypotension is recommended. For paralysis succinylcholine or rocuronium can be used. Recommendations for post-intubation continuous sedation medications include a combination of propofol and fentanyl in the normotensive or hypertensive patient. A combination of midazolam and fentanyl or ketamine alone should be considered in the hypotensive patient. Delayed sequence induction (DSI) or a ketamine-only intubation, in which ketamine is used without a paralytic are very promising options for emergency intubation and may become the standard of care in the future. The benefit of these strategies compared to RSI need to be confirmed in large randomized clinical trials.

Acknowledgements

We thank Clerc EMS Monthey, Switzerland for providing **Figure 1**.

Conflict of interest

The authors declare no conflict of interest.

Author details

Dominik A. Jakob[1,2], Jean-Cyrille Pitteloud[3] and Demetrios Demetriades[1]*

1 Division of Trauma and Surgical Critical Care, Department of Surgery, Los Angeles County + University of Southern California Medical Center, University of Southern California, Los Angeles, CA, USA

2 Department of Surgical Emergency Unit, Inselspital University of Bern, Bern, Switzerland

3 Hospital du Jura Bernois, Saint-Imier, Switzerland

*Address all correspondence to: demetrios.demetriades@med.usc.edu

References

[1] Henry SM. American College of Surgeons Committee on Trauma. Student course manual ATLS ® Advanced Trauma Life Support ®. 10th edn. Chicago, IL; 2018

[2] Mayglothling J, Duane TM, Gibbs M, McCunn M, Legome E, Eastman AL, et al. Emergency tracheal intubation immediately following traumatic injury: An Eastern Association for the Surgery of Trauma practice management guideline. Journal of Trauma and Acute Care Surgery. 2012;**73**(5 Suppl. 4):S333-S340. DOI: 10.1097/TA.0b013e31827018a5

[3] Jakob DA, Lewis M, Benjamin ER, Demetriades D. Isolated traumatic brain injury: Routine intubation for Glasgow Coma Scale 7 or 8 may be harmful! Journal of Trauma and Acute Care Surgery. 2021;**90**(5):874-879. DOI: 10.1097/TA.0000000000003123

[4] Oestern HJ, Trentz O, Uranues S. General trauma care and related aspects: Trauma surgery II. New York, NY: Springer; 2013

[5] Choi J, Carlos G, Nassar AK, Knowlton LM, Spain DA. The impact of trauma systems on patient outcomes. Current Problems in Surgery. 2021;**58**(1):100849. DOI: 10.1016/j.cpsurg.2020.100849

[6] Badjatia N, Carney N, Crocco TJ, Fallat ME, Hennes HM, Jagoda AS, et al. Guidelines for prehospital management of traumatic brain injury 2nd edition. Prehospital Emergency Care. 2008;**12**(Suppl. 1):S1-S52. DOI: 10.1080/10903120701732052

[7] Spaite DW, Bobrow BJ, Keim SM, Barnhart B, Chikani V, Gaither JB, et al. Association of statewide implementation of the prehospital traumatic brain injury treatment guidelines with patient survival following traumatic brain injury: The excellence in prehospital injury care (EPIC) study. JAMA Surgery. 2019;**154**(7):e191152. DOI: 10.1001/jamasurg.2019.1152

[8] Broderick ED, Sauerberg N, Reed JJ. EMS Pros And Cons Of Drug-Assisted Intubation. Treasure Island (FL): StatPearls; 2022

[9] Pepe PE, Roppolo LP, Fowler RL. Prehospital endotracheal intubation: Elemental or detrimental? Critical Care. 2015;**19**:121. DOI: 10.1186/s13054-015-0808-x

[10] Teasdale G, Maas A, Lecky F, Manley G, Stocchetti N, Murray G. The Glasgow Coma Scale at 40 years: Standing the test of time. Lancet Neurology. 2014;**13**(8):844-854. DOI: 10.1016/S1474-4422(14)70120-6

[11] Rotheray KR, Cheung PS, Cheung CS, Wai AK, Chan DY, Rainer TH, et al. What is the relationship between the Glasgow coma scale and airway protective reflexes in the Chinese population? Resuscitation. 2012;**83**(1):86-89. DOI: 10.1016/j.resuscitation.2011.07.017

[12] Haltmeier T, Schnuriger B, Benjamin E, Brodmann Maeder M, Kunzler M, Siboni S, et al. Isolated blunt severe traumatic brain injury in Bern, Switzerland, and the United States: A matched cohort study. Journal of Trauma and Acute Care Surgery. 2016;**80**(2):296-301. DOI: 10.1097/TA.0000000000000892

[13] Davis DP, Peay J, Sise MJ, Vilke GM, Kennedy F, Eastman AB, et al. The

impact of prehospital endotracheal intubation on outcome in moderate to severe traumatic brain injury. The Journal of Trauma. 2005;**58**(5):933-939. DOI: 10.1097/01.ta.0000162731.53812.58

[14] Davis DP, Fakhry SM, Wang HE, Bulger EM, Domeier RM, Trask AL, et al. Paramedic rapid sequence intubation for severe traumatic brain injury: Perspectives from an expert panel. Prehospital Emergency Care. 2007;**11**(1):1-8. DOI: 10.1080/10903120601021093

[15] Davis DP, Peay J, Serrano JA, Buono C, Vilke GM, Sise MJ, et al. The impact of aeromedical response to patients with moderate to severe traumatic brain injury. Annals of Emergency Medicine. 2005;**46**(2):115-122. DOI: 10.1016/j.annemergmed.2005.01.024

[16] Gamberini L, Giugni A, Ranieri S, Meconi T, Coniglio C, Gordini G, et al. Early-onset ventilator-associated pneumonia in severe traumatic brain injury: Is there a relationship with prehospital airway management? The Journal of Emergency Medicine. 2019;**56**(6):657-665. DOI: 10.1016/j.jemermed.2019.02.005

[17] Bernard SA, Nguyen V, Cameron P, Masci K, Fitzgerald M, Cooper DJ, et al. Prehospital rapid sequence intubation improves functional outcome for patients with severe traumatic brain injury: A randomized controlled trial. Annals of Surgery. 2010;**252**(6):959-965. DOI: 10.1097/SLA.0b013e3181efc15f

[18] Warner KJ, Cuschieri J, Copass MK, Jurkovich GJ, Bulger EM. The impact of prehospital ventilation on outcome after severe traumatic brain injury. The Journal of Trauma. 2007;**62**(6):1330-1336, discussion 6-8. DOI: 10.1097/TA.0b013e31804a8032

[19] Carney N, Totten AM, Cheney T, Jungbauer R, Neth MR, Weeks C, et al. Prehospital airway management: A systematic review. Prehospital Emergency Care. 2021:1-12. DOI: 10.1080/10903127.2021.1940400

[20] Hatchimonji JS, Dumas RP, Kaufman EJ, Scantling D, Stoecker JB, Holena DN. Questioning dogma: Does a GCS of 8 require intubation? European Journal of Trauma and Emergency Surgery. 2021;**47**(6):2073-2079. DOI: 0.1007/s00068-020-01383-4

[21] Muakkassa FF, Marley RA, Workman MC, Salvator AE. Hospital outcomes and disposition of trauma patients who are intubated because of combativeness. The Journal of Trauma. 2010;**68**(6):1305-1309. DOI: 10.1097/TA.0b013e3181dcd137

[22] Tong JL, Ashworth DR, Smith JE. Cardiovascular responses following laryngoscope assisted, fibreoptic orotracheal intubation. Anaesthesia. 2005;**60**(8):754-758. DOI: 10.1111/j.1365-2044.2005.04238.x

[23] Robinson N, Clancy M. In patients with head injury undergoing rapid sequence intubation, does pretreatment with intravenous lignocaine/lidocaine lead to an improved neurological outcome? A review of the literature. Emergency Medicine Journal. 2001;**18**(6):453-457. DOI: 10.1136/emj.18.6.453

[24] Svedung Wettervik T, Howells T, Hillered L, Nilsson P, Engquist H, Lewen A, et al. Mild hyperventilation in traumatic brain injury-relation to cerebral energy metabolism, pressure autoregulation, and clinical outcome. World Neurosurgery. 2020;**133**:e567-ee75. DOI: 10.1016/j.wneu.2019.09.099

[25] Cook AM, Morgan Jones G, Hawryluk GWJ, Mailloux P, McLaughlin D, Papangelou A, et al. Guidelines for the acute treatment of cerebral edema in neurocritical care patients. Neurocritical Care. 2020;**32**(3):647-666. DOI: 10.1007/s12028-020-00959-7

[26] Langeron O, Birenbaum A, Amour J. Airway management in trauma. Minerva Anestesiologica. 2009;**75**(5):307-311

[27] Stept WJ, Safar P. Rapid induction-intubation for prevention of gastric-content aspiration. Anesthesia and Analgesia. 1970;**49**(4):633-636

[28] Sakles JC, Chiu S, Mosier J, Walker C, Stolz U. The importance of first pass success when performing orotracheal intubation in the emergency department. Academic Emergency Medicine. 2013;**20**(1):71-78. DOI: 10.1111/acem.12055

[29] Root CW, Mitchell OJL, Brown R, Evers CB, Boyle J, Griffin C, et al. Suction assisted laryngoscopy and airway decontamination (SALAD): A technique for improved emergency airway management. Resuscitation Plus. 2020;**1-2**:100005. DOI: 10.1016/j.resplu.2020.100005

[30] Davis DP, Hwang JQ, Dunford JV. Rate of decline in oxygen saturation at various pulse oximetry values with prehospital rapid sequence intubation. Prehospital Emergency Care. 2008;**12**(1):46-51. DOI: 10.1080/10903120701710470

[31] Green SM, Roback MG, Kennedy RM, Krauss B. Clinical practice guideline for emergency department ketamine dissociative sedation: 2011 update. Annals of Emergency Medicine. 2011;**57**(5):449-461. DOI: 10.1016/j.annemergmed.2010.11.030

[32] Hudetz JA, Pagel PS. Neuroprotection by ketamine: A review of the experimental and clinical evidence. Journal of Cardiothoracic and Vascular Anesthesia. 2010;**24**(1):131-142. DOI: 10.1053/j.jvca.2009.05.008

[33] Kramer N, Lebowitz D, Walsh M, Ganti L. Rapid sequence intubation in traumatic brain-injured adults. Cureus. 2018;**10**(4):e2530. DOI: 10.7759/cureus.2530

[34] Tran DT, Newton EK, Mount VA, Lee JS, Wells GA, Perry JJ. Rocuronium versus succinylcholine for rapid sequence induction intubation. Cochrane Database of Systematic Reviews. 2015;**10**:CD002788. DOI: 10.1002/14651858.CD002788.pub3

[35] Weingart SD, Trueger NS, Wong N, Scofi J, Singh N, Rudolph SS. Delayed sequence intubation: A prospective observational study. Annals of Emergency Medicine. 2015;**65**(4):349-355. DOI: 10.1016/j.annemergmed.2014.09.025

[36] Merelman AH, Perlmutter MC, Strayer RJ. Alternatives to rapid sequence intubation: Contemporary airway management with ketamine. The Western Journal of Emergency Medicine. 2019;**20**(3):466-471. DOI: 10.5811/westjem.2019.4.42753

Chapter 3

Neuroinflammation in Traumatic Brain Injury

Grace Y. Kuo, Fawaz Philip Tarzi, Stan Louie and Roy A. Poblete

Abstract

Neuroinflammation following traumatic brain injury (TBI) is an important cause of secondary brain injury that perpetuates the duration and scope of disease after initial impact. This chapter discusses the pathophysiology of acute and chronic neuroinflammation, providing insight into factors that influence the acute clinical course and later functional outcomes. Secondary injury due to neuroinflammation is described by mechanisms of action such as ischemia, neuroexcitotoxicity, oxidative stress, and glymphatic and lymphatic dysfunction. Neurodegenerative sequelae of inflammation, including chronic traumatic encephalopathy, which are important to understand for clinical practice, are detailed by disease type. Prominent research topics of TBI animal models and biomarkers of traumatic neuroinflammation are outlined to provide insight into the advances in TBI research. We then discuss current clinical treatments in TBI and their implications in preventing inflammation. To complete the chapter, recent research models, novel biomarkers, and future research directions aimed at mitigating TBI will be described and will highlight novel therapeutic targets. Understanding the pathophysiology and contributors of neuroinflammation after TBI will aid in future development of prophylaxis strategies, as well as more tailored management and treatment algorithms. This topic chapter is important to both clinicians and basic and translational scientists, with the goal of improving patient outcomes in this common disease.

Keywords: neuroinflammation, traumatic brain injury, inflammatory cytokines, metabolomics and lipidomics, blood-brain barrier, ischemia, neuronal excitotoxicity, chronic traumatic encephalopathy

1. Introduction

Traumatic brain injury (TBI) remains a significant source of morbidity, mortality and increased global healthcare burden and costs. Even among survivors and those classified as having mild TBI, outcomes are often poor [1–3]. This highlights the need for continued research into understanding the pathophysiology of disease and its association with clinical outcomes.

Secondary injury after TBI is exacerbated by several biochemical processes post trauma, including inflammation [4]. Through the neuroinflammatory cascade, traumatic injuries affect brain structure and function far beyond the acute phase, resulting in heterogeneity of TBI outcomes [5, 6]. Although the primary intent for the inflammatory response is tissue repair, collateral damage can occur if left unregulated and sustained [7]. Animal models have demonstrated that targeting neuroinflammation can alter the biologic process of injury. Unfortunately, effective pharmacological strategies to decrease inflammation in vitro still have not translated into benefit in clinical trials. Continuing research and understanding of neuroinflammation in TBI will provide important guidance into future prognostication methods and therapeutic targets.

2. The pathophysiology of inflammation

While trauma such as blunt force, penetrating injury, or shearing energy, causes the primary injury in TBI, secondary injury can occur in delayed fashion. Pathologic processes that underlie secondary brain injury can persist for days to years after the initial trauma. Neuroinflammation following TBI is a principal driver of secondary injury and is characterized by complex intercellular signaling and profound histochemical changes.

2.1 The acute neuroinflammatory response

Tissue and neuronal injury occurring after trauma activates the release of danger signals. Also known as damage-associated molecular pattern molecules (DAMPs), these trigger an innate immune response and inflammasome activation [6, 8]. Various intracellular molecules can act as DAMPs, including DNA, RNA, high mobility group box 1 (HMGB1), S100 proteins, adenosine triphosphate (ATP), uric acid, lysophospholipids, and lipid peroxidation-derived carbonyl adducts of proteins [9]. Early cytokines are released in damaged tissues within minutes of trauma which typically peak within the first 24 hours [6]. A classic DAMP is HMGB1, which signals through toll-like receptors 2 (TLR-2) and 4 (TLR-4) to increase cytokine production and release [8, 10]. HMGB1, a nuclear protein present in all cell types, attaches onto TLR-4 and activates the NLRP3 inflammasome complex, priming it for further inflammation in response to stressors. The activated inflammasome complex cleaves cytokine precursors such as pro-IL1ß and pro-caspase to create its active metabolite [10].

Responding to early DAMPs release, activated microglia with a pro-inflammatory phenotype release additional cytokines into the extracellular space, potentiating the neuroinflammatory response [3]. Tumor necrosis factor (TNF), and interleukins (ILs) are two primary inflammatory cytokines implicated in neuroinflammation. In animal models, an increase in IL-1β expression is seen as early as 1 hour after trauma [11, 12]. Similarly, increased TNF levels are observed in brain tissue within 17 minutes of injury in a murine model [13]; however, correlation between early cytokine levels and functional outcomes has been conflicting [6]. Studies have not been able to correlate TNF levels with raised ICPs and poor neurological outcomes [14]; TNF levels are also not a good predictor of additional neuronal injury in the immediate hours post injury [15]. Chemokines such as CXCL8 and chemoattractant molecules like CCL2 are observed to be increased in response to cytokines such as IL-1B and TNF, which are elevated after brain injury, and associated with neurological deficit after ischemia [16–19]. Further studies of these cytokines and their role in predicting TBI outcomes are still necessary to elucidate their clinical utility.

Apart from microglia, several other resident central nervous system (CNS) immune cells are capable of expressing cytokines to regulate post-traumatic inflammation. Neutrophils are the earliest and most abundant immune cells to enter the CNS in response to chemokines, with natural killer (NK) cells, dendritic cells and T-lymphocytes also being observed but in less abundance [8, 20]. Matrix metalloproteinases (MMPs) and reactive oxygen species (ROS) are released by neutrophils to promote cellular repair; but, in the acute post-traumatic milieu, these molecules potentiate the breakdown of the blood brain barrier (BBB), promoting migration of immune cells into the CNS, and can lead to delayed secondary hemorrhagic complications after trauma [8, 9]. Within the CNS, astrocyte activity increases within the first few days after injury, undergoing reactive gliosis. Glial fibrillary acidic protein (GFAP) is subsequently upregulated and cytokine production is increased [21]. Highlighting the importance of the inflammatory cascade in mediating secondary brain injury, GFAP levels have been correlated with clinical outcomes in TBI patients [22], and may serve as a biomarker for disease severity.

2.2 The role of chronic neuroinflammation in traumatic brain injury pathology

In addition to the acute and subacute post-trauma inflammatory response, TBI survivors are prone to the development of chronic neuroinflammation that persists for years after injury [8, 23–25]. How acute inflammation transitions to a chronic pro-inflammatory state is not fully understood. Mouse models of TBI have shown that cortical inflammation persists even 30 days post injury and is associated with increased microglial activity [26, 27]. In contrast, mice with genetically depleted microglia did not display the same level of inflammatory response as their wild type counterparts, suggesting the central role of microglia in establishing chronic inflammation [28]. Microglial dysfunction and increased white matter phagocytosis is also associated with chronic neuroinflammation in TBI survivors [23]. Imaging studies in rat TBI models have demonstrated a persistent increase in BBB permeability up to 10 months post injury, and an elevation in CD68, a marker for activated microglia and macrophages, in perilesional cortical tissue up to 11 months post injury [29]. These findings suggest that monocyte extravasation from the blood and into the CNS are capable of sustaining chronic inflammation.

Chronic neuroinflammation may also involve activation of systemic inflammation. Effects of post-traumatic microglial activation can also be observed in regions distant to the brain [24, 28]. Macrophage biomarker studies have also shown chronically elevated serum TNF levels after TBI, with increased TNF levels being associated with unfavorable behavioral outcomes [30]. Plasma levels of pro-inflammatory chemokines and cytokines including interferon gamma (IFN-γ), TNF, IL-8, IL-17A, IL-9, eotaxin, macrophage inflammatory protein-1-beta (MIP-1β), and monocyte chemoattractant protein 1 (MCP-1) remain elevated for over 12 months even in patients with mild TBI with normal magnetic resonance imaging (MRI) brain imaging [31]. Chronic inflammation of both the CNS and systemically likely contributes to long-term neuropsychiatric and poor functional outcomes in post-TBI survivors and those with chronic traumatic encephalopathy (CTE). Ongoing research and expert opinion further implicate long-term systemic inflammation as underlying the etiology psychiatric, neurologic, cardiovascular, renal and liver disease, as well as cancer and metabolic syndrome (**Figure 1**) [32, 33].

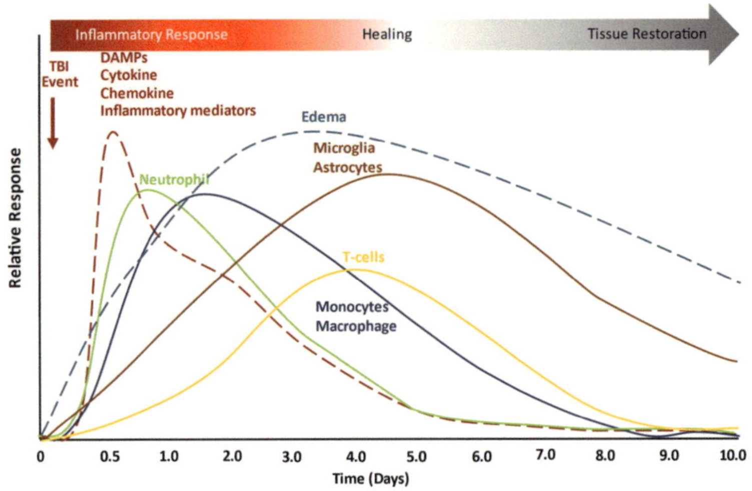

Figure 1.
Timeline of neuroinflammation post-TBI.

3. Mechanisms of secondary brain injury mediated by neuroinflammation

Following TBI, primary injury occurs at the time of trauma as a direct result of the force transferred to the head and brain tissue. This leads to contusion, vascular injury, and axonal shearing. Secondary brain injury results from a complex TBI pathophysiology that leads to extensive and persistent neurologic structural and functional changes. While primary injury is considered irreversible, secondary brain injury is hypothetically preventable. As neuroinflammation is a central mediator of secondary brain injury, it is an important target for research and therapeutic development. Here, we describe primary pathologic processes that are associated with neuroinflammation after TBI.

3.1 Increased blood-brain barrier permeability

The BBB is formed by tightly connected cerebrovascular endothelial cells supported by astrocyte foot processes, pericytes, and basement membrane. It is highly regulated and functions as the interface between peripheral circulation and the CNS. Loss of BBB integrity after brain injury can contribute to neuronal cell death and affect the brain's response to pharmacologic therapy. The underlying structural changes leading to increased BBB permeability following TBI are not fully elucidated. Brain injury has been associated with an increase in the numbers of endothelial caveolae, leading to an increase in transcytosis of plasma proteins and a decrease in the expression of junctional adhesion and tight junction proteins [34, 35]. Under ischemic conditions, BBB integrity may be lost independent of tight junctions and occurs following endothelial swelling and disruption of the basement membrane [36, 37].

The breakdown of the BBB has been strongly linked to inflammation. Within tight junctions, upregulation of vascular endothelial growth factor-A (VEGF-A) from neutrophils and astrocytes act to reduce the expression of tight junction protein claudin-5, leading to BBB leakage [38]. In pro-inflammatory states, activated microglia and recruited neutrophils can sequester in the tissues and elaborate a network of DNA, MMPs, proteases and eicosanoids which is referred to as neutrophil extracellular traps (a process commonly termed NETosis). NETotic neutrophils release MMPs and neutrophil elastase (NE) that contribute to degradation of the extracellular matrix [39]. In parallel, microglia promote the expression of Aquaporin-4 (AQP-4), contributing to fluid shifts into the CNS [40].

Once BBB integrity is lost, the influx of peripheral neutrophils, macrophages, natural killer cells, T helper cells, and cytotoxic T cells intended to facilitate tissue repair can sustain neuroinflammation, BBB permeability, and promote secondary brain injury. Elevations of these immune cells and other inflammatory mediators are measurable following human TBI [41, 42]. Extravasation of albumin and other plasma proteins also contribute to the activation of microglia and astrocytes to trigger the release cytokines, chemokines and MMPs [41]. The formation of ROS is associated with MMP activation, resulting in further tissue damage and BBB disruption [43]. Tissue debris from both primary and secondary brain injury contain DNA, RNA, proteins and lipids that can activate TLRs and exacerbate neuroinflammation. These findings highlight the ability of inflammation to be self-propagating and dependent on BBB permeability.

The clinical impact of BBB disruption after TBI is profound. Cerebral edema is the major clinical consequence of BBB dysfunction and occurs due to the increased permeability of the BBB to protein-rich fluid and neuroinflammatory cells into the extracellular space leading to interstitial edema [38]. Cerebral edema is often symptomatic, can lead to increased intracranial pressure and reduced cerebral perfusion and oxygenation, and can be life-threatening when it results in brain compression and herniation.

3.2 Ischemia and tissue hypoxia

Ischemia and hypoxia occur after TBI for several reasons that include intracranial hypertension, reduced cerebral perfusion pressures, and abnormal cerebral autoregulation that result in the inadequate supply of oxygen-rich blood to vulnerable brain regions [44]. Independent of hemodynamics, tissue-mediated clotting and neuroinflammation promote microcirculatory failure and increased ischemic burden that may go clinically unrecognized. Neuroinflammation can directly contribute to microvascular disruption by causing endothelial dysfunction. Functionally, endothelial-dependent vasodilation is diminished after TBI due to impaired nitric oxide (NO) production from uncoupling of endothelial nitric oxide synthase (NOS) [45]. Additionally, reduced capacity for oxygen diffusion due to endothelial cell edema leads to diminished levels of brain oxygen tension in CNS tissue after TBI [46]. Structurally, the activation of MMPs and increased oxidative stress leads to the degradation of vascular basement membrane proteins which results in endothelium instability and loss of cellular integrity [47].

Other factors promote hypoxia and ischemia during neuroinflammation. Neuronal death from cellular hypoxia causes the release of pro-inflammatory cytokines and chemokines. Excess neutrophil activation exacerbates inflammation and competes with neurons for limited oxygen [48]. During NETosis, neutrophil pseudopods that adhere to the endovascular endothelium hinder microcirculatory function and further promote hypoperfusion and neutrophils adherence. Additionally, hypoxic events after TBI induce hypoxia-inducible factor -1a and nuclear factor kappa B (NF-kB) leading to prolongation of neutrophil survival time and activation [49].

The clinical implications of ischemia and tissue hypoxia are significant. A large portion of TBI patients experience ischemic-hypoxic injury [50]; however, the real ischemic burden in TBI is likely underestimated. Anoxic brain injury following TBI is strongly associated with worse functional outcomes [51]. Ischemic burden, therefore, may be an important intermediate surrogate of disease in TBI research.

3.3 Neuroexcitotoxicity and energy dysfunction

Neuroexcitotoxicity and disrupted energetics after TBI potentiate neuroinflammatory cascades. At injury onset, mechanical stretching of neurons elicits glutamate-independent neuronal activation, inhibiting the magnesium blockade of calcium channels on the cell membrane. In this environment, neurons and glial cells transition into an excessively neuroexcitatory state [52]. Secondary brain injury ensues if reduced cerebral perfusion or ischemia occur in the setting of increased metabolic demand.

Glutamate-dependent pathways are the primary drivers of neuroexcitotoxicity. Glutamate, the most abundant excitatory neurotransmitter of the CNS, contributes to the excitotoxic milieu and is released in large amounts after neuron lysis [8, 53, 54]. Animal models demonstrate an increased extracellular glutamate concentration post-trauma due to altered glutamate transport receptor function and concentration [55, 56]. The acute elevation in glutamate levels overwhelm NMDA and AMPA receptors, exacerbating neuronal injury and death. Ultimately, an influx of calcium into the cell activates apoptosis [57]. Apart from cellular effects, NMDA receptor activation induces inflammatory gene expression. Additionally, TNF and IL-1ß glutamate transporters on astrocytes interfere with glutamate clearance; together, this creates sustained excitotoxicity and inflammation [58].

The post-trauma brain is also affected by disturbed ionic homeostasis and increased energy demands from post-injury repair mechanisms. Microdialysate studies in clinical and experimental TBI models have shown increases in interstitial lactate, adenosine and a concurrent decrease in glucose, consistent with a state of metabolic crisis [59, 60]. Murine TBI models have demonstrated that both acute and delayed changes in energy metabolism occur. Increased glucose consumption and decreased ATP availability were observed on days 1 and 3 post-trauma [61]. Furthermore, mitochondrial fission is disrupted after TBI, contributing to the inability of neurons and glial cells to meet metabolic needs [62].

3.4 Oxidative stress

Oxidative stress describes a state where oxygen-derived free radicals overwhelm the scavenging antioxidant system and is closely related to metabolic dysfunction. Ischemia is an important trigger that promotes anaerobic metabolism and cellular acidosis that activates pH-dependent calcium channels [63]. Decreased cytoplasmic pH triggers increased ROS production which is ultimately involved in lipid peroxidation. Proton extrusion by microglia further exacerbates extracellular acidosis seen in TBI [64].

Post-TBI oxidative stress is regulated by microglia. Following brain injury, microglia activate nicotinamide adenine dinucleotide phosphate oxidase (NOX) and inducible nitric oxide synthase (iNOS). Upregulation of iNOS leads to the production of NO, which when coupled with superoxide, leads to the formation of peroxynitrite. The damaging role of peroxynitrite has been shown indirectly by the ability of peroxynitrite-derived free radical scavengers to attenuate brain injury in TBI [65]. NOX is present in other neuroinflammatory cells such as neutrophils and phagocytic cells, contributing to oxidative stress through the production of superoxide and hydroxyl radicals [66].

ROS will directly target mitochondria, impair ATP synthesis and lead to secondary injury [67]. Additionally, calcium overload in CNS mitochondria will disrupt fusion and fission, two important mechanisms essential in mitochondrial function. This promotes additional free radical formation [68]. Mitochondrial dysfunction due to oxidative stress results in functional impairment and is associated with reduced neuronal repair. Oxidative stress occurs even in mild TBI [69], with ongoing pre-clinical research investigating the effectiveness of anti-oxidant therapy in TBI [70].

3.5 Glymphatic and lymphatic dysfunction

The glymphatic system is a complex transport system that facilitates the exchange of cerebrospinal (CSF) and interstitial fluid by aiding the movement of water, metabolites and immune molecules [71]. Facilitated by AQP-4 channels, glymphatics provide a drainage route for CSF and aid in the surveillance of the CNS by carrying macromolecules and activated antigen-bearing dendritic cells to local lymph nodes where antigens can be presented to activate the adaptive immune response.

TBI and neuroinflammation have been shown to impair glymphatic system drainage. In animal models, TBI dramatically impairs the paravascular influx of CSF MRI tracer, especially in the ipsilateral cortex [72]. A > 25% reduction in glymphatic solute clearance is observed after TBI [73]. Glymphatic function is dependent on AQP-4 channels localized on astrocytes. TBI-induced damage to AQP4 channels contributes glymphatic dysfunction [74]. Re-localization of AQP4 channels away from astrocytic end feet is associated with reduced waste and immune cell clearance [75, 76]. In addition to glymphatics, CNS clearance is also facilitated by lymphatic vessels lining the dura and meningeal vessels. These are rich in T and B cells that readily migrate to injured brain region [77].

Failure of glymphatic and lymphatic function will lead to the accumulation of damage and waste products such as tau, beta-amyloid, pro-inflammatory mediators, and astrocytic proteins [74]. Glial scar formation and reactive astrogliosis may also

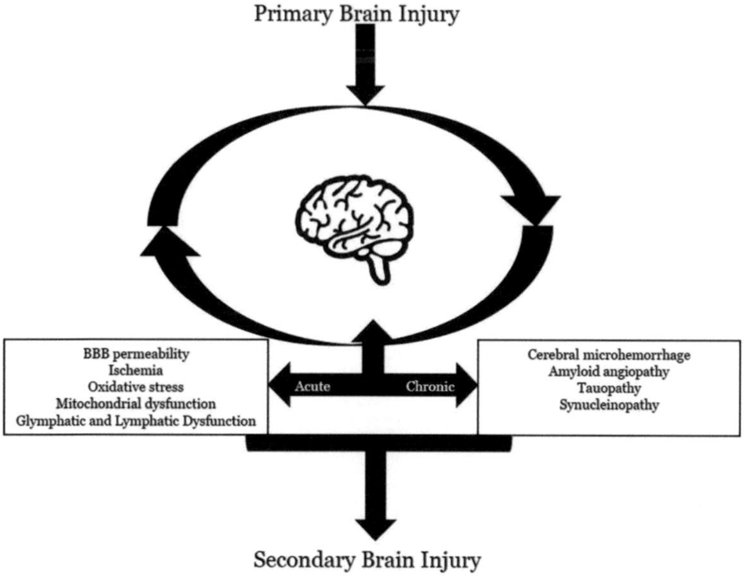

Figure 2.
Conceptual schematic of neuroinflammatory Cascade.

occur [73]. The accumulation of both immune cells and waste products triggers further neuroinflammation by activation of pattern recognition receptors on microglia. These cells and peptides have an important role in the development of neurofibrillary tangle pathology and neurodegeneration in secondary brain injury and the development of CTE (**Figure 2**) [73].

4. Neurodegeneration and long-term sequelae of neuroinflammation

Neurodegeneration and chronic symptomatology occur in survivors of both single and repeated TBI, such as military personnel and contact sport athletes. Progressive symptoms long after trauma has been described as early as the 1920s [78], but the underlying pathogenesis is complex. Recent advances in research implicate chronic inflammation in the development of post-TBI neurodegenerative disease. Autopsy investigation of those who survive >1 year after TBI revealed increased amounts of CNS microglia compared to control tissue [24, 79]. Similarly, positron emission tomography (PET) imaging of professional football players showed greater levels of microglia compared to age-matched controls [80]. Here, we describe distinct pathological and clinical findings that are associated with chronic inflammation following TBI.

4.1 Cerebral microhemorrhage and amyloid angiopathy

The presence of cerebral microhemorrhage is often an indicator of traumatic axonal injury [81, 82]. Older TBI patients are particularly at risk of developing cerebral microbleeds post-TBI due to the senescent BBB having a higher permeability exacerbated by chronic neuroinflammation [83]. Cerebral amyloid angiopathy (CAA) is also a risk factor for microhemorrhage formation, as amyloid accumulation in the vessel walls, especially in the elderly, make them prone to rupture [84, 85]. Apolipoprotein E4 (ApoE4), an important regulator of chronic neuroinflammation, might play a central role. The ApoE4 allele predisposes later development of CAA in TBI survivors [86]. Further study is needed to elucidate the specific mechanism that ApoE4-mediated neuroinflammation results in CAA.

Trauma-induced microhemorrhage and CAA can occur in younger populations, especially with repetitive trauma. In a study of sport-related repetitive head trauma, athletes participating in high-risk sports had increased CAA burden in the frontal and leptomeningeal regions compared to a control population [87]. Microhemorrhage and CAA is seen in TBI survivors in their second and third decades [86, 88]. Since CAA is often a post-mortem diagnosis, the causality of trauma on CAA is still under investigation. Recently, animal models have demonstrated that increased transforming growth factor (TGF-β) expression is associated with the development of CAA after TBI [89].

4.2 Dementia and other neurodegenerative diseases after brain trauma

Early population studies have linked TBI to cognitive decline in both Alzheimer's dementia (AD) and non-Alzheimer's dementia [90–93]. More recent epidemiologic analysis suggests that TBI is significantly associated with dementia, but not AD specifically [90].

Amyloid beta (Aβ) and tau-induced inflammation are important in the pathogenesis of neurodegenerative disease. A rat TBI model demonstrated that progressive atrophy and neuronal cell death continues >1 year after the trauma [94]. PET imaging studies have shown increased Aβ deposition after TBI [95]. Neuroinflammation plays a role in the pathogenesis of tau accumulation [96]. Both acute and chronic activation of the innate immune system exacerbates tau phosphorylation [96–98]. In a rat model of chronic inflammation, implantation of slow-release IL-1β pellets was associated with increased tau phosphorylation [99]. Knocking out receptors that suppress microglial activation results in an enhanced neuroinflammatory response and tau phosphorylation [100]. Conversely, immune suppression is associated with a reduction of p-tau [101]. Anti-inflammatory medications such as infliximab, an TNF-α antagonist, also reduced levels of p-tau in murine models [102]; however, in vitro application of TNF-α and IL-6 did not increase tau levels [103, 104]. Further investigation is needed to better understand the mechanisms by which inflammation after TBI promotes tau pathology.

Parkinson-like symptoms also occur after trauma, suggesting a potential α-synucleinopathy in chronic TBI survivors [105, 106]. Scientific evidence for the importance of α-synuclein pathology is less robust compared to Aβ and tauopathies. Murine models have demonstrated an increase in α-synuclein accumulation in the substantia nigra ipsilateral to the trauma. Furthermore, a notable upregulation of inflammatory cells was observed in the substantia nigra and cerebral peduncles, suggesting that inflammation mediates alpha-synucleinopathies post TBI [105].

4.3 Neuroinflammation in chronic traumatic encephalopathy

Chronic traumatic encephalopathy is a syndrome of neuropsychiatric, cognitive and motor deterioration after repeated exposure to head trauma. Pathologically, CTE is a tauopathy characterized by perivascular accumulation of p-tau in neurons and astrocytes within the cortex [107]. As previously described, neuroinflammation is involved in the formation of p-tau. Immunohistologic analysis of samples from the Boston University-VA Concussion Legacy Foundation Brain Bank showed that a longer history of repeated head injury was associated with increased neuroinflammation [108]. CTE genetic transcripts from brain tissue contain dysregulated neuronal genes that result in inflammatory glial dysfunction. Furthermore, CTE astrocytes express gene transcripts that were associated with neuroinflammation and aging [109]. Autopsy investigation of mild CTE brain tissue revealed increased microglia activation in perivascular regions of subcortical white matter [106, 110, 111]. In vivo diagnostics of National Football League (NFL) athletes utilizing PET imaging revealed an increase in translocator protein expression by activated microglia and reactive astrocytes compared to controls [80, 95]. Further research is needed to elucidate the pathway and time course of inflammation and development of CTE, as well as genetic and epigenetic risk factors that increases the likelihood of CTE after head trauma.

5. Animal models of post-injury neuroinflammation

The initiation and propagation of neuroinflammation is a complex and multifaceted process. Animal models are necessary to study disease mechanisms, identify novel biomarkers, and study the pharmacologic effects of investigational drugs. Given the current limited treatment options in TBI management, translational research should prioritize research that is validated, feasible and most readily will impact patient care.

5.1 Selection of animals

Several animal models have been used in TBI research. Interspecies differences in cerebral anatomy, complexity, and size are important factors when selecting the model. Animal intelligence varies significantly, although brain size is not correlated with overall intelligence [112]. Most preclinical TBI research is conducted in rodents. Rats and mice are cost-effective, have a large physiological database, permit extensive behavioral testing and have the ability to utilize transgenic animals. A disadvantage is the small lissencephalic brain, characterized by less white matter compared with higher species. In particular, the utilization of genetically engineered mice has aided in the evaluation of key molecules related to microglia activation and neuroinflammation following TBI [26].

More recently, the use of large animals in TBI research has increased. The effect of brain injury on lissencephalic animals as compared to larger ones with gyrencephalic structures differ, at least in part by differences in brain structure and mechanics related to the presence of large gyri [113, 114]. The porcine model has been proposed as an ideal pre-clinical animal model based on feasibility and the anatomic and physiologic similarities to humans in comparison to rodents [115]. This includes cortical structure and proportion of gray-to-white matter that more closely resembles humans [116]. Both mild and more severe TBI can be modeled in the pig.

5.2 Models of injury

Several models of injury have been developed to resemble the pathophysiology of human TBI [113]. The most used ones are the lateral fluid percussion (LFP) model, the controlled cortical impact (CCI) model, the weight drop-impact (WD) model, and the blast model. The chosen mechanism of injury is based on researcher experience and the type of TBI being modeled. Traumatic injury can be delivered over an intact skull to mimic concussion or diffuse injury or delivered to exposed dura to mimic more severe and focal TBI.

The CCI model was first described in the 1980s and is now one of the most used TBI models. It utilizes a pneumatic or electromechanical device with an impactor tip to induce brain displacement. The impact location, velocity, depth, and dwell time can be controlled. Compared to other methods of mechanical injury, namely LFP and WD injury, CCI allows for more control of the force of injury, showing high reproducibility, low animal mortality, and reduced rebound injury [117]. Current CCI rodent models produce the most optimal conditions for understanding the molecular, cellular and biochemical mechanisms of secondary brain injury after focal blunt-force TBI [118].

The WD and LFP models are also used to study neuroinflammation. In WD injury, a fixed amount of weight is dropped from a set height onto either exposed dura or closed skull. The closed-head model can be utilized to cause diffuse neuronal injury and has been shown to result in elevation of apoptotic and neuroinflammatory markers. The LFP model was first established in rabbit and cat models but has since been adapted for rodents. It involves the generation of a fluid pulse that impacts against an exposed dural surface of the brain and produces more diffuse injury compared to CCI. Reproducibility requires extensive preparation and model experience to minimize injury variability. The blast model mimics the injuries commonly encountered in war. The force is produced by utilizing shockwave tubes or open field detonation. This model has been utilized to study CTE and its associated neuroinflammation [119].

6. Biomarkers of neuroinflammation

Plasma biomarkers of post-TBI inflammation are commonly used in translational research given their accessibility, the ability to serially sample, the presence of validated assays for detection, and the ability to form large biorepositories and databases. Brain tissue and CSF biosamples can be difficult to obtain but may offer a more accurate picture of the local environment. There has been growing interest in identifying and validating in vivo markers of neuroinflammation with special focus on using functional MRI and PET to measure intermediate biomarkers of disease.

The number of biomarkers of neuroinflammation studied is rapidly increasing [26]. No gold standard biomarker has been established. Understanding the mechanisms of expression of these markers will advance our understanding of TBI and help develop future therapeutics targeting the acute and chronic consequences of neuroinflammation. Here, we aim to introduce biomarkers of importance and emerging interest in the field of post-TBI neuroinflammation and discuss potential limitations.

6.1 Peptide biomarkers

Peptide cytokines are the most used biomarkers of inflammation. In the acute period, TBI induces damage to the cellular membrane, leading to the release of DAMPs and upregulation of TNF-α and other cytokines from microglia and astrocytes. Historically, the cytokines most studied include INF-γ and several ILs. There are important limitations to consider when using cytokine biomarkers. Changes in cytokine expression can be non-specific, and their relationship with clinical outcomes is variable. TNF-α is generally considered a pro-inflammatory cytokine associated with detrimental effects in TBI [120, 121]; however, studies have suggested that it also has an anti-inflammatory component that promotes motor recovery after TBI [122]. Several studies have found limited correlation between ILs such as IL-1β and IL-6 and outcome in human TBI [123, 124]. Chemokines, generated by activated microglia and astrocytes to recruit peripheral immune cells to the site of injury, can also be assayed from biofluids. The CCL and CXCL subclasses of chemokines have been most extensively characterized in animal models of post-TBI inflammation [26]. The expression of cytokines and chemokines is regulated several ways; therefore, measurements may provide a general description of the inflammatory response post-TBI but might lack the specificity in describing specific biochemical pathways or differentiating between CNS and systemic inflammation.

More novel peptide biomarkers of interest include neurotransmitter levels and protein aggregates. Post-TBI, a large increase in the release of extracellular glutamate and other amino acids can be studied. Glutamate is an excitatory amino acid that can lead to toxic effects via activation of different receptors such as N-methyl-D-aspartate (NMDA) and alpha-amino-3-hydroxy-5-methyl-4-isoxazole propionic acid receptors (AMPA) [53, 54]. In clinical research, glutamate can be measured longitudinally using bedside microdialysis techniques [125]. Protein aggregates such as Aβ, tau and α-synuclein are challenging to measure. Historically, they have been limited to post-mortem analysis; however, recent advances in PET imaging have allowed in vivo assessment of tau burden [126].

6.2 Glial and immune cells

Microglial activation and neutrophil recruitment and activation have been of principle interest in post-TBI neuroinflammation research. Common immunohistochemical measures of microglial activation include Iba-1 and CD68 and downstream markers such as TLRs and NF-kβ [26, 127]; however, flow cytometry-based analysis of microglia remains the gold standard. The identification of translocator protein 18 kDa (TSPO), located on the mitochondrial membrane of microglia, has allowed the development of radioligands with PET visualization of activated microglia in vivo [128].

Activated neutrophils and NETosis are measured commonly by TLR4 expression, CitH3 localization, and DNase-I expression, which acts to degrade neutrophil-derived extracellular traps [129]. Measures of endothelial adhesion molecules including selectins, vascular cell adhesion molecules (VCAMs), and intercellular adhesion molecules (ICAMs) provide an indirect measurement of peripheral immune cell recruitment across the BBB. Antibodies against several of these adhesion molecules have been developed and utilized for in vivo visualization by MRI but is mostly validated in ischemic stroke models [130–132]. The longitudinal study of glial and immune cell phenotypes in chronic post-TBI inflammation may further demonstrate their importance mediating long-term morbidity after brain injury.

6.3 Omics-based biomarkers

Multi-omics, including genomics, proteomics, metabolomics and lipidomics can be used to characterize the complex chemical pathways involved in TBI pathogenesis for use in prediction models and drug development. Genetic analysis can elucidate the genetic influence on post-TBI outcomes and would allow precision treatment based on genetic traits. In analysis of a large biologic database, genetic modules that showed greatest change in expression were primarily associated with neurodevelopment and immune inflammation [133]. As previously discussed, the ApoE-4 allele is also of special interest in the field of chronic TBI-induced inflammation. ApoE protein is a mediator of cholesterol and lipid transport in the brain and has been shown to attenuate glial activation and CNS inflammatory responses. In experimental models, a small peptide of ApoE [133–149] was shown to significantly improve histological and functional outcomes following TBI [134].

Lipid biomarker analysis might hold several advantages over proteomics and peptide biomarkers in TBI. Limitations of proteomics include a bias towards highly abundant proteins, difficulty in measuring protein aggregates, and challenges in using plasma samples to assay proteins generated in the CNS [135]. In comparison, lipids are abundant in the CNS and cross the BBB by active transport. Bioactive lipids that mediate inflammation are of particular interest due to their role in both pro-inflammatory cell signaling and resolution of inflammation. Omega-3 polyunsaturated fatty acids (ω-3 PUFAs), including eicosatetraenoic acid and docosahexaenoic acid, are active compounds with anti-neuroinflammatory properties. In pro-inflammatory states, they are metabolized by lipoxygenases (e.g. 15-LOX and 5-LOX) to specialized pro-resolving lipid mediators (SPMs) such as resolvins, protectins, and maresins. In experimental models, ω-3 PUFAs act as a neuroprotectant in TBI by modulating neuroinflammation through SIRT1 mediated deacetylation of the HMGB1/NF-kb pathway [136]. A greater understanding of the biologic actions of SPMs and other lipid signaling molecules, and the mechanisms of lipid metabolism dysregulation related to TBI would identify novel therapeutic targets.

7. Current therapies with anti-inflammatory properties

Attenuating neuroinflammation following TBI has been a treatment target for several decades to generally mixed results. Certain current standard treatments potentially work through anti-inflammatory pathways, while neuroinflammation remains a focus for novel therapeutic development.

7.1 Steroidal and non-steroidal anti-inflammatory drugs

Steroids are not routinely used in the management of TBI. They were initially investigated for their potential to decrease neuroinflammation and intracranial pressure in severe TBI. Several randomized trials were conducted with conflicting results. The CRASH trial, a randomized placebo-controlled multicentric trial evaluated the use of high dose methylprednisolone after TBI. Interim analysis of the first 10,008 patients demonstrated increased mortality in patients receiving steroids, resulting in early study closure [137]. The mechanisms of harm are not fully understood; however, there is little interest in a future study of the effect of high-dose steroids in TBI.

The use of non-steroidal anti-inflammatory drugs (NSAIDs), such as COX-1 and COX-2 inhibitors ibuprofen and indomethacin, have shown varied results in pre-clinical studies. Although a strong anti-inflammatory action is observed if dosed shortly before or after injury, clinical effect has not been demonstrated [138]. Ibuprofen can cross the BBB and localize in injured tissues and has been studied as an anti-inflammatory agent in post-TBI stem cell grafting [139]. In a rat model of TBI, extended use of high dose ibuprofen significantly worsened neurocognitive outcomes [140]. Indomethacin administration is associated with reduced intracranial pressure secondary to reduced CBF [141], however, it has limited therapeutic potential due to its inability to cross the BBB [142]. Additional concerns over bleeding due to inhibition of platelet cyclooxygenase further limit their use acutely after TBI.

Minocycline, a second-generation tetracycline antibiotic, has been extensively studied in TBI due to its anti-inflammatory, neuroprotective and anti-apoptotic properties [143]. In a murine model, minocycline administration resulted in marked reductions of activated microglia and decreased tissue IL-1B levels [144]. In a gerbil model, when administered shortly after ischemia, minocycline was neuroprotective against brain ischemia by preventing activation of microglia and the appearance of NADPH reactive cells [145]. A clinical trial of 15 patients, performed to assess the safety and feasibility of minocycline showed that it was safe for moderate-to-severe TBI with a potential effect on clinical outcomes [146]; however, long-term use may be associated with gastrointestinal and neurologic adverse events [147]. The current use of minocycline is limited due to the lack of large longitudinal clinical evidence to support its use for TBI-related neuroinflammation.

7.2 Anti-epileptic drugs

Seizures are a common consequence of TBI. Their occurrence is associated with worse functional outcomes and if uncontrolled, can contribute to long-term neurodegeneration [148]. Neuroinflammation has been proposed as a mechanistic cause of seizures post-TBI. Pro-inflammatory cytokines like TNF-α and IL-1β can lead to hyperexcitability through their action on glutamate and NMDA receptors, increasing susceptibility to seizures [149]. Classical anti-epileptics such as phenytoin and benzodiazepines have not been shown to reduce the risk of developing late post-traumatic epilepsy but rather decrease the early post-traumatic seizures occurring within the first 7 days [150]. Whether anti-epileptic drugs are generally pro-inflammatory or anti-inflammatory is still not verified. Levetiracetam interestingly has been found to mediate its anti-epileptogenic effects, at least partially, through modulation of inflammation in seizing brain regions. This was demonstrated by the reduction of reactive gliosis and IL-1β following administration of levetiracetam in epileptic animals [151]. In comparison, an in vitro model of epilepsy showed increased microglial activation in cultures treated with valproic acid when compared to carbamazepine, gabapentin, and phenytoin [152].

7.3 Hyperosmolar fluids

Hyperosmolar therapy is widely used to treat TBI-related cerebral edema and elevated intracranial pressure. The early action is primarily due to the creation of an osmotic gradient that draws interstitial fluid from the brain tissue into the intravascular space. Hyperosmolar therapies, typically hypertonic saline or mannitol, have been investigated for their anti-inflammatory properties. In a rat model of intracerebral hemorrhage, hyperosmolar fluid reduced microglial activation and promoted phagocytic anti-inflammatory M2-like phenotype in perihematomal and contralateral tissues [153]. In a clinical study of 65 patients with severe TBI, hypertonic saline was found to attenuate expression of pro-inflammatory cytokines such as TNF-α and IL-10 [154]. Additionally, hyperosmolar therapy was found to downregulate AQP-4 expression in perivascular astrocytes [155]. These findings add further support to hyperosmolar therapy for their neuroinflammatory modulation.

In clinical practice, bolus doses of hyperosmolar therapy are standard of care for clinical or radiographic cerebral herniation; however, the use of continuous hypertonic saline infusion after TBI remains controversial with a recent randomized controlled trial showing no benefit of this therapy on 6-month functional outcomes [156]. Further study is needed to determine the anti-inflammatory properties of hyperosmolar therapy, and which patients are most likely to benefit from treatment.

7.4 Tranexamic acid

Tranexamic acid (TXA) is a lysine analogue that is widely studied as an anti-fibrinolytic in life-threatening hemorrhage. In TBI, TXA is more widely accepted and used based on recent clinical trial data. The CRASH 3 trial demonstrated that TXA reduces head injury-related deaths without increasing the thrombotic risk [157]. TXA has been shown to have both pro-inflammatory and anti-inflammatory effects in the surgical literature [158, 159]. In animal models, it inhibits plasmin which normally activates the migration of macrophages through modulation of BBB integrity by degrading laminin, fibronectin, and collagen [160]. Specifically in models of TBI, early TXA has been shown to reduce TBI-induced coagulopathy. Reduced bleeding and blood products in the CNS might limit pro-inflammatory triggering. TXA may generally suppress circulating immune cells; however, measurable reductions in anti-inflammatory markers were not observed in a mouse model of TBI [161]. Although

TXA is approved to be safe and well-studied in TBI, its full impact on neuroinflammation has not been validated.

7.5 Hypothermia

Hypothermia has been investigated in several acute neurological conditions. In TBI, humoral and cellular neuroinflammation is temperature-dependent. In preclinical trials, hypothermia has been shown to decrease free radicals, TNF-α mRNA levels, and BBB permeability [162]. Several clinical trials of hypothermia have been done in TBI, with overall low-quality evidence. A meta-analysis in 2014 suggested a possible trend towards reduced rates of death, vegetative state, and disability with hypothermia [163]; however, the report was inconclusive. Larger clinical trials are needed to assess the efficacy and safety of hypothermia in reducing neuroinflammation in TBI and improving clinical outcomes.

8. Future research directions

Advances in novel therapies that target neuroinflammation after TBI has been limited by an incomplete understanding of the pathologic mechanisms of disease. Translational and clinical research is needed to further identify both modifiable and non-modifiable factors that influence the inflammatory response, and how acute neuroinflammation after brain injury transitions to a chronic inflammatory state. Characterizing both acute and chronic processes will lead to biomarker discovery and support the development of novel therapeutic agents aimed at improving long-term patient outcomes.

8.1 Determining how biologic factors modify the inflammatory response post-injury

Non-modifiable biologic factors such as age, sex, and ethnicity likely influence the post-TBI inflammatory response. A better understanding of these effects will improve patient-tailored treatments. In animal models, age appears to exacerbate inflammatory-mediated secondary brain injury. In comparison to younger animals, aged rodents show higher mortality after CCI, more pronounced brain edema formation, and worse neurobehavioral scores [164]. This was associated with an early rise of inflammatory markers in aged animals compared to the delayed response observed in younger mice. Peripherally derived CCR2(+) macrophages accumulate in greater amounts in aged brains after TBI compared to young animals and likely mediate the enhanced neuroinflammatory response associated with age [165]; however, the role of other immune cells has been suggested [166]. Ketone metabolism, which improves energetics and reduces inflammation, is reduced in older age [167, 168]. Additional research is necessary to fully describe the age-dependent effects of TBI and how age influences the efficacy of candidate drugs.

Although the majority of TBI occurs in males, sex-based differences in TBI pathophysiology and outcomes should be understood. Elevations in endogenous sex hormones, specifically progesterone and allopregnanolone, have been demonstrated to have anti-inflammatory and neuroprotective properties [169]. Sex steroids are also known to regulate astrogliosis and microglia activation and may account for sex differences [170]. Investigational drugs, including steroids, likely have differential impact in men and women, highlighting the need to study efficacy in diverse patient populations. Although many identified differences in physiology between sexes exist, the literature of the impact of sex on functional outcomes after TBI is conflicting [171].

8.2 Important research questions for novel therapeutic approaches

Despite the large body of anti-inflammatory drugs studied in both preclinical and clinical research [172], their standard use in human TBI has not yet been supported by high-quality evidence. Many important questions remain, including the identification of drugs that should be prioritized for clinical trials. Candidate drugs or anti-inflammatory drug classes may not be mutually exclusive and could have a synergistic effect when used together. In animal models, combination of progesterone and vitamin D, fresh frozen plasma and valproic acid, and C3a and C5a receptor blockers demonstrated greater anti-inflammatory and neuroprotective effects then when used individually [173–175]. The optimal timing and duration of potential treatments are also unknown. Given both the acute and chronic inflammatory phases of TBI contribute to functional outcomes, future study is needed to determine the utility of anti-inflammatory drugs administered beyond the acute phase.

Both short and long-term outcome measures are necessary to establish the efficacy of novel therapies. In pre-clinical research, measures of inflammatory cytokines are insufficient to characterize the complex pathogenesis of TBI. Of emerging interest, use of "omics" that encompass genomics, proteomics, metabolomics and lipidomics will provide a comprehensive picture of the molecular pathways leading to secondary brain injury and would allow for precision medicine [176]. Given the chronic morbidity in TBI survivors, the use of long-term outcomes, including biomarkers of neurodegeneration and neurocognitive and functional outcomes are needed in both animal models and clinical trials. Demonstrating reduced mortality in TBI can be difficult, especially in moderate-to-severe TBI where outcomes are generally poor, while alternative outcome measures described may be more sensitive and meaningful.

TBI is a ubiquitous disease impacting all ages, genders, racial, socioeconomic and geographic backgrounds. Preferred drug therapies should be safe, feasible and effective across mixed patient populations and medical environments. Behavioral modifications may play a role in attenuating sequelae of neuroinflammation. Complementary therapies such as meditation and massage may reduce inflammation [177], while dietary changes can also impact chronic inflammation [178, 179]. Ultimately, a multi-disciplinary and systems-based approach to TBI is needed to further our understanding of this challenging disease and promote the development of novel treatment approaches.

8.3 Conclusion

In conclusion, post-TBI neuroinflammation is a complex blend of processes that is involved in acute and chronic brain injury. Although it is intended to promote repair, ongoing neuroinflammation can impede recovery. The inflammatory cascade in TBI affects the CNS milieu and brain functions long after the initial traumatic phase. Although pre-clinical research suggests that treating neuroinflammation as a therapeutic target may be beneficial, clinical trials have not yielded measurable benefits. Understanding the intricacy of these processes will assist clinicians and scientists in creating an individualistic approach to monitor and limit inflammation after TBI with the goal to reduce secondary brain injury, enhance neurological repair, and improve patient outcomes.

Author details

Grace Y. Kuo[1*], Fawaz Philip Tarzi[1], Stan Louie[2] and Roy A. Poblete[1]

1 Department of Neurology, Keck School of Medicine of the University of Southern California, United States

2 Department of Clinical Pharmacy, University of Southern California School of Pharmacy, United States

*Address all correspondence to: grace.kuo@med.usc.edu

References

[1] CDC. TBI Data | Concussion | Traumatic Brain Injury | CDC Injury Center. 2021. Available from: https://www.cdc.gov/traumaticbraininjury/data/index.html

[2] Haarbauer-Krupa J, Pugh MJ, Prager EM, Harmon N, Wolfe J, Yaffe K. Epidemiology of chronic effects of traumatic brain injury. Journal of Neurotrauma. 2021;**38**(23):3235-3247

[3] Xiong Y, Mahmood A, Chopp M. Current understanding of neuroinflammation after traumatic brain injury and cell-based therapeutic opportunities. Chinese Journal of Traumatology. 2018;**21**(3):137-151

[4] Jassam YN, Izzy S, Whalen M, McGavern DB, El Khoury J. Neuroimmunology of traumatic brain injury: Time for a paradigm shift. Neuron. 2017;**95**(6):1246-1265

[5] Pagulayan KF, Temkin NR, Machamer J, Dikmen SS. A longitudinal study of health-related quality of life after traumatic brain injury. Archives of Physical Medicine and Rehabilitation. 2006;**87**(5):611-618

[6] Woodcock T, Morganti-Kossmann MC. The role of markers of inflammation in traumatic brain injury. Frontiers in Neurology. 2013;**4**:18

[7] Finnie JW. Neuroinflammation: Beneficial and detrimental effects after traumatic brain injury. Inflammopharmacology. 2013;**21**(4):309-320

[8] Simon DW, McGeachy M, Bayır H, Clark RSB, Loane DJ, Kochanek PM. Neuroinflammation in the evolution of secondary injury, repair, and chronic neurodegeneration after traumatic brain injury. Nature Reviews Neurology. 2017;**13**(3):171-191

[9] Corps KN, Roth TL, McGavern DB. Inflammation and neuroprotection in traumatic brain injury. JAMA Neurology. 2015;**72**(3):355-362

[10] Frank MG, Weber MD, Watkins LR, Maier SF. Stress sounds the alarmin: The role of the danger-associated molecular pattern HMGB1 in stress-induced neuroinflammatory priming. Brain, Behavior, and Immunity. 2015;**48**:1-7

[11] Fan L, Young PR, Barone FC, Feuerstein GZ, Smith DH, McIntosh TK. Experimental brain injury induces expression of interleukin-1 beta mRNA in the rat brain. Brain Research. Molecular Brain Research. 1995;**30**(1):125-130

[12] Kamm K, Vanderkolk W, Lawrence C, Jonker M, Davis AT. The effect of traumatic brain injury upon the concentration and expression of interleukin-1beta and interleukin-10 in the rat. The Journal of Trauma. 2006;**60**(1):152-157

[13] Frugier T, Morganti-Kossmann MC, O'Reilly D, McLean CA. In situ detection of inflammatory mediators in post mortem human brain tissue after traumatic injury. Journal of Neurotrauma. 2010;**27**(3):497-507

[14] Shiozaki T, Hayakata T, Tasaki O, Hosotubo H, Fuijita K, Mouri T, et al. Cerebrospinal fluid concentrations of anti-inflammatory mediators in early-phase severe traumatic brain injury. Shock. 2005;**23**(5):406-410

[15] Hayakata T, Shiozaki T, Tasaki O, Ikegawa H, Inoue Y, Toshiyuki F, et al. Changes in CSF S100B and cytokine concentrations in early-phase severe traumatic brain injury. Shock. 2004;**22**(2):102-107

[16] Kasahara T, Mukaida N, Yamashita K, Yagisawa H, Akahoshi T, Matsushima K. IL-1 and TNF-alpha induction of IL-8 and monocyte chemotactic and activating factor (MCAF) mRNA expression in a human astrocytoma cell line. Immunology. 1991;**74**(1):60-67

[17] Semple BD, Kossmann T, Morganti-Kossmann MC. Role of chemokines in CNS health and pathology: A focus on the CCL2/CCR2 and CXCL8/CXCR2 networks. Journal of Cerebral Blood Flow and Metabolism. 2010;**30**(3):459-473

[18] Taupin V, Toulmond S, Serrano A, Benavides J, Zavala F. Increase in IL-6, IL-1 and TNF levels in rat brain following traumatic lesion. Influence of pre- and post-traumatic treatment with Ro5 4864, a peripheral-type (p site) benzodiazepine ligand. Journal of Neuroimmunology. 1993;**42**(2):177-185

[19] Chen Y, Hallenbeck JM, Ruetzler C, Bol D, Thomas K, Berman NE, et al. Overexpression of monocyte chemoattractant protein 1 in the brain exacerbates ischemic brain injury and is associated with recruitment of inflammatory cells. Journal of Cerebral Blood Flow and Metabolism. 2003;**23**(6):748-755

[20] Clark RS, Schiding JK, Kaczorowski SL, Marion DW, Kochanek PM. Neutrophil accumulation after traumatic brain injury in rats: Comparison of weight drop and controlled cortical impact models. Journal of Neurotrauma. 1994;**11**(5):499-506

[21] Burda JE, Bernstein AM, Sofroniew MV. Astrocyte roles in traumatic brain injury. Experimental Neurology. 2016;**275**(Pt 3):305-315

[22] Wang KK, Yang Z, Zhu T, Shi Y, Rubenstein R, Tyndall JA, et al. An update on diagnostic and prognostic biomarkers for traumatic brain injury. Expert Review of Molecular Diagnostics. 2018;**18**(2):165-180

[23] Gentleman SM, Leclercq PD, Moyes L, Graham DI, Smith C, Griffin WST, et al. Long-term intracerebral inflammatory response after traumatic brain injury. Forensic Science International. 2004;**146**(2-3):97-104

[24] Johnson VE, Stewart JE, Begbie FD, Trojanowski JQ, Smith DH, Stewart W. Inflammation and white matter degeneration persist for years after a single traumatic brain injury. Brain (London, England : 1878). 2013;**136**(Pt 1):28-42

[25] Ramlackhansingh AF, Brooks DJ, Greenwood RJ, Bose SK, Turkheimer FE, Kinnunen KM, et al. Inflammation after trauma: Microglial activation and traumatic brain injury. Annals of Neurology. 2011;**70**(3):374-383

[26] Chiu C-C, Liao Y-E, Yang L-Y, Wang J-Y, Tweedie D, Karnati HK, et al. Neuroinflammation in animal models of traumatic brain injury. Journal of Neuroscience Methods. 2016;**272**:38-49

[27] Loane DJ, Kumar A, Stoica BA, Cabatbat R, Faden AI. Progressive neurodegeneration after experimental brain trauma: Association with chronic microglial activation. Journal of Neuropathology and Experimental Neurology. 2014;**73**(1):14-29

[28] Witcher KG, Bray CE, Chunchai T, Zhao F, O'Neil SM, Gordillo AJ, et al. Traumatic brain injury causes chronic cortical inflammation and neuronal dysfunction mediated by microglia. The Journal of Neuroscience. 2021;**41**(7):1597-1616

[29] van Vliet EA, Ndode-Ekane XE, Lehto LJ, Gorter JA, Andrade P, Aronica E, et al. Long-lasting blood-brain barrier dysfunction and neuroinflammation after traumatic brain injury. Neurobiology of Disease. 2020;**145**:105080

[30] Juengst SB, Kumar RG, Arenth PM, Wagner AK. Exploratory associations with tumor necrosis factor-α, disinhibition and suicidal endorsement after traumatic brain injury. Brain, Behavior, and Immunity. 2014;**41**:134-143

[31] Chaban V, Clarke GJB, Skandsen T, Islam R, Einarsen CE, Vik A, et al. Systemic inflammation persists the first year after mild traumatic brain injury: Results from the prospective trondheim mild traumatic brain injury study. Journal of Neurotrauma. 2020;**37**(19):2120-2130

[32] Bauer ME, Teixeira AL. Inflammation in psychiatric disorders: What comes first? Annals of the New York Academy of Sciences. 2019;**1437**(1):57-67

[33] Furman D, Campisi J, Verdin E, Carrera-Bastos P, Targ S, Franceschi C, et al. Chronic inflammation in the etiology of disease across the life span. Nature Medicine. 2019;**25**(12):1822-1832

[34] Nag S, Manias JL, Stewart DJ. Expression of endothelial phosphorylated caveolin-1 is increased in brain injury. Neuropathology and Applied Neurobiology. 2009;**35**(4):417-426

[35] Yeung D, Manias JL, Stewart DJ, Nag S. Decreased junctional adhesion molecule—A expression during blood–brain barrier breakdown. Acta Neuropathologica. 2008;**115**(6):635-642

[36] Krueger M, Bechmann I, Immig K, Reichenbach A, Hartig W, Michalski D. Blood-brain barrier breakdown involves four distinct stages of vascular damage in various models of experimental focal cerebral ischemia. Journal of Cerebral Blood Flow and Metabolism. 2015;**35**(2):292-303

[37] Krueger M, Hartig W, Reichenbach A, Bechmann I, Michalski D. Blood-brain barrier breakdown after embolic stroke in rats occurs without ultrastructural evidence for disrupting tight junctions. PLoS One. 2013;**8**(2):e56419

[38] Argaw AT, Gurfein BT, Zhang Y, Zameer A, John GR. VEGF-mediated disruption of endothelial CLN-5 promotes blood-brain barrier breakdown. Proceedings of the National Academy of Sciences. 2009;**106**(6):1977-1982

[39] Yang H, Biermann MH, Brauner JM, Liu Y, Zhao Y, Herrmann M. New insights into neutrophil extracellular traps: Mechanisms of formation and role in inflammation. Frontiers in Immunology. 2016;**7**:302

[40] Neri M, Frati A, Turillazzi E, Cantatore S, Cipolloni L, Di Paolo M, et al. Immunohistochemical evaluation of Aquaporin-4 and its correlation with CD68, IBA-1, HIF-1alpha, GFAP, and CD15 expressions in fatal traumatic brain injury. International Journal of Molecular Sciences. 2018;**19**(11):3544

[41] Corrigan F, Mander KA, Leonard AV, Vink R. Neurogenic inflammation after traumatic brain injury and its

potentiation of classical inflammation. Journal of Neuroinflammation. 2016;**13**(1):264

[42] Holmin S, Söderlund J, Biberfeld P, Mathiesen T. Intracerebral inflammation after human brain contusion. Neurosurgery. 1998;**42**(2):291-298

[43] Ranaivo HR, Hodge JN, Choi N, Wainwright MS. Albumin induces upregulation of matrix metalloproteinase-9 in astrocytes via MAPK and reactive oxygen species-dependent pathways. Journal of Neuroinflammation. 2012;**9**(1):645

[44] Rangel-Castilla L, Gasco J, Nauta HJW, Okonkwo DO, Robertson CS. Cerebral pressure autoregulation in traumatic brain injury. Neurosurgical Focus. 2008;**25**(4):E7-EE

[45] Villalba N, Sackheim AM, Nunez IA, Hill-Eubanks DC, Nelson MT, Wellman GC, et al. Traumatic brain injury causes endothelial dysfunction in the systemic microcirculation through Arginase-1-dependent uncoupling of endothelial nitric oxide synthase. Journal of Neurotrauma. 2017;**34**(1):192-203

[46] Schilte C, Bouzat P, Millet A, Boucheix P, Pernet-Gallay K, Lemasson B, et al. Mannitol improves brain tissue oxygenation in a model of diffuse traumatic brain injury. Critical Care Medicine. 2015;**43**(10):2212-2218

[47] Abdul-Muneer PM, Chandra N, Haorah J. Interactions of oxidative stress and neurovascular inflammation in the pathogenesis of traumatic brain injury. Molecular Neurobiology. 2015;**51**(3):966-979

[48] Liu Y-W, Li S, Dai S-S. Neutrophils in traumatic brain injury (TBI): Friend or foe? Journal of Neuroinflammation. 2018;**15**(1):146

[49] Walmsley SR, Print C, Farahi N, Peyssonnaux C, Johnson RS, Cramer T, et al. Hypoxia-induced neutrophil survival is mediated by HIF-1α–dependent NF-κB activity. Journal of Experimental Medicine. 2005;**201**(1):105-115

[50] Padayachy LC, Rohlwink U, Zwane E, Fieggen G, Peter JC, Figaji AA. The frequency of cerebral ischemia/hypoxia in pediatric severe traumatic brain injury. Child's Nervous System. 2012;**28**(11):1911-1918

[51] Cullen NK, Crescini C, Bayley MT. Rehabilitation outcomes after anoxic brain injury: A case-controlled comparison with traumatic brain injury. PM&R. 2009;**1**(12):1069-1076

[52] Tehse J, Taghibiglou C. The overlooked aspect of excitotoxicity: Glutamate-independent excitotoxicity in traumatic brain injuries. European Journal of Neuroscience. 2019;**49**(9):1157-1170

[53] Palmer AM, Marion DW, Botscheller ML, Bowen DM, DeKosky ST. Increased transmitter amino acid concentration in human ventricular CSF after brain trauma. Neuroreport. 1994;**6**(1):153-156

[54] Ruppel RA, Kochanek PM, Adelson PD, Rose ME, Wisniewski SR, Bell MJ, et al. Excitatory amino acid concentrations in ventricular cerebrospinal fluid after severe traumatic brain injury in infants and children: The role of child abuse. The Journal of Pediatrics. 2001;**138**(1):18-25

[55] Dorsett CR, McGuire JL, Niedzielko TL, DePasquale EAK, Meller J, Floyd CL, et al. Traumatic brain injury induces alterations in cortical glutamate uptake without a reduction in glutamate

transporter-1 protein expression. Journal of Neurotrauma. 2017;**34**(1):220-234

[56] Pajarillo E, Rizor A, Lee J, Aschner M, Lee E. The role of astrocytic glutamate transporters GLT-1 and GLAST in neurological disorders: Potential targets for neurotherapeutics. Neuropharmacology. 2019;**161**:107559

[57] Baracaldo-Santamaría D, Ariza-Salamanca DF, Corrales-Hernández MG, Pachón-Londoño MJ, Hernandez-Duarte I, Calderon-Ospina C-A. Revisiting excitotoxicity in traumatic brain injury: From bench to bedside. Pharmaceutics. 2022;**14**(1):152

[58] Viviani B, Boraso M, Marchetti N, Marinovich M. Perspectives on neuroinflammation and excitotoxicity: A neurotoxic conspiracy? Neurotoxicology. 2014;**43**:10-20

[59] Faroqi AH, Lim MJ, Kee EC, Lee JH, Burgess JD, Chen R, et al. In vivo detection of extracellular adenosine triphosphate in a mouse model of traumatic brain injury. Journal of Neurotrauma. 2021;**38**(5):655-664

[60] Marklund N, Salci K, Ronquist G, Hillered L. Energy metabolic changes in the early post-injury period following traumatic brain injury in rats. Neurochemical Research. 2006;**31**(8):1085-1093

[61] Buczek M, Alvarez J, Azhar J, Zhou Y, Lust WD, Selman WR, et al. Delayed changes in regional brain energy metabolism following cerebral concussion in rats. Metabolic Brain Disease. 2002;**17**(3):153-167

[62] Fischer TD, Hylin MJ, Zhao J, Moore AN, Waxham MN, Dash PK. Altered mitochondrial dynamics and TBI pathophysiology. Frontiers in Systems Neuroscience. 2016;**10**:29

[63] Angeloni C, Prata C, Vieceli Dalla Sega F, Piperno R, Hrelia S. Traumatic brain injury and NADPH oxidase: A deep relationship. Oxidative Medicine and Cellular Longevity. 2015;**2015**:1-10

[64] Ritzel RM, He J, Li Y, Cao T, Khan N, Shim B, et al. Proton extrusion during oxidative burst in microglia exacerbates pathological acidosis following traumatic brain injury. Glia. 2021;**69**(3):746-764

[65] Deng-Bryant Y, Singh IN, Carrico KM, Hall ED. Neuroprotective effects of tempol, a catalytic scavenger of peroxynitrite-derived free radicals, in a mouse traumatic brain injury model. Journal of Cerebral Blood Flow & Metabolism. 2008;**28**(6):1114-1126

[66] Cooney SJ, Bermudez-Sabogal SL, Byrnes KR. Cellular and temporal expression of NADPH oxidase (NOX) isotypes after brain injury. Journal of Neuroinflammation. 2013;**10**(1):917

[67] Uzhachenko R, Boyd K, Olivares-Villagomez D, Zhu Y, Goodwin JS, Rana T, et al. Mitochondrial protein Fus1/Tusc2 in premature aging and age-related pathologies: Critical roles of calcium and energy homeostasis. Aging. 2017;**9**(3):627-649

[68] Magenta A, Dellambra E, Ciarapica R, Capogrossi MC. Oxidative stress, microRNAs and cytosolic calcium homeostasis. Cell Calcium. 2016;**60**(3):207-217

[69] Petronilho F, Feier G, de Souza B, Guglielmi C, Constantino LS, Walz R, et al. Oxidative stress in brain according to traumatic brain injury intensity. The Journal of Surgical Research. 2010;**164**(2):316-320

[70] Hakiminia B, Alikiaii B, Khorvash F, Mousavi S. Oxidative stress and mitochondrial dysfunction

following traumatic brain injury: From mechanistic view to targeted therapeutic opportunities. Fundamental & Clinical Pharmacology. 2022;**36**(4):612-662

[71] Rasmussen MK, Mestre H, Nedergaard M. The glymphatic pathway in neurological disorders. The Lancet Neurology. 2018;**17**(11):1016-1024

[72] Yang L, Kress BT, Weber HJ, Thiyagarajan M, Wang B, Deane R, et al. Evaluating glymphatic pathway function utilizing clinically relevant intrathecal infusion of CSF tracer. Journal of Translational Medicine. 2013;**11**(1):107

[73] Iliff JJ, Chen MJ, Plog BA, Zeppenfeld DM, Soltero M, Yang L, et al. Impairment of glymphatic pathway function promotes tau pathology after traumatic brain injury. The Journal of Neuroscience. 2014;**34**(49):16180-16193

[74] Iliff JJ, Wang M, Liao Y, Plogg BA, Peng W, Gundersen GA, et al. A paravascular pathway facilitates CSF flow through the brain parenchyma and the clearance of interstitial solutes, including amyloid β. Science Translational Medicine. 2012;**4**(147):147ra111

[75] Iliff JJ, Lee H, Yu M, Feng T, Logan J, Nedergaard M, et al. Brain-wide pathway for waste clearance captured by contrast-enhanced MRI. Journal of Clinical Investigation. 2013;**123**(3):1299-1309

[76] Taoka T, Masutani Y, Kawai H, Nakane T, Matsuoka K, Yasuno F, et al. Evaluation of glymphatic system activity with the diffusion MR technique: Diffusion tensor image analysis along the perivascular space (DTI-ALPS) in Alzheimer's disease cases. Japanese Journal of Radiology. 2017;**35**(4):172-178

[77] Utagawa A, Truettner JS, Dietrich WD, Bramlett HM. Systemic inflammation exacerbates behavioral and histopathological consequences of isolated traumatic brain injury in rats. Experimental Neurology. 2008;**211**(1):283-291

[78] Faden AI, Loane DJ. Chronic neurodegeneration after traumatic brain injury: Alzheimer disease, chronic traumatic encephalopathy, or persistent neuroinflammation? Neurotherapeutics. 2014;**12**(1):143-150

[79] Smith C, Gentleman SM, Leclercq PD, Murray LS, Griffin WS, Graham DI, et al. The neuroinflammatory response in humans after traumatic brain injury. Neuropathology and Applied Neurobiology. 2013;**39**(6):654-666

[80] Coughlin JM, Wang Y, Minn I, Bienko N, Ambinder EB, Xu X, et al. Imaging of glial cell activation and white matter integrity in brains of active and recently retired national football league players. JAMA Neurology. 2017;**74**(1):67-74

[81] Glushakova OY, Johnson D, Hayes RL. Delayed increases in microvascular pathology after experimental traumatic brain injury are associated with prolonged inflammation, blood-brain barrier disruption, and progressive white matter damage. Journal of Neurotrauma. 2014;**31**(13):1180-1193

[82] Liu J, Kou Z, Tian Y. Diffuse axonal injury after traumatic cerebral microbleeds: An evaluation of imaging techniques. Neural Regeneration Research. 2014;**9**(12):1222-1230

[83] Irimia A, Van Horn JD, Vespa PM. Cerebral microhemorrhages due to traumatic brain injury and their effects on the aging human brain. Neurobiology of Aging. 2018;**66**:158-164

[84] Dada MA, Rutherfoord GS. Medicolegal aspects of cerebral amyloid angiopathy. A case report. The American Journal of Forensic Medicine and Pathology. 1993;**14**(4):319-322

[85] Wakui K, Seguchi K, Kuroyanagi T, Sakai T, Tanaka Y, Kamijoh Y, et al. Multiple intracerebral hemorrhages due to cerebral amyloid angiopathy after head trauma. No Shinkei Geka. 1988;**16**(11):1287-1291

[86] Leclercq PD, Murray LS, Smith C, Graham DI, JaR N, Gentleman SM. Cerebral amyloid angiopathy in traumatic brain injury: Association with apolipoprotein E genotype. Journal of Neurology, Neurosurgery, and Psychiatry. 2005;**76**(2):229-233

[87] Standring OJ, Friedberg J, Tripodis Y, Chua AS, Cherry JD, Alvarez VE, et al. Contact sport participation and chronic traumatic encephalopathy are associated with altered severity and distribution of cerebral amyloid angiopathy. Acta Neuropathologica. 2019;**138**(3):401-413

[88] Nakayama Y, Mineharu Y, Arawaka Y, Nishida S, Tsuji H, Miyake H, et al. Cerebral amyloid angiopathy in a young man with a history of traumatic brain injury: A case report and review of the literature. Acta Neurochirurgica. 2016;**159**(1):15-18

[89] Wyss-Coray T, Masliah E, Mallory M, McConlogue L, Johnson-Wood K, Lin C, et al. Amyloidogenic role of cytokine TGF-beta1 in transgenic mice and in Alzheimer's disease. Nature. 1997;**389**(6651):603-606

[90] Wang H-K, Lin S-H, Sung P-S, Wu M-H, Hung K-W, Wang L-C, et al. Population based study on patients with traumatic brain injury suggests increased risk of dementia. Journal of Neurology, Neurosurgery, and Psychiatry. 2012;**83**(11):1080-1085

[91] Mortimer JA, van Duijn CM, Chandra V, Fratiglioni L, Graves AB, Heyman A, et al. Head trauma as a risk factor for Alzheimer's disease: A collaborative re-analysis of case-control studies. EURODEM risk factors research group. International Journal of Epidemiology. 1991;**20**(Suppl. 2):S28-S35

[92] Guo Z, Cupples LA, Kurz A, Auerbach SH, Volicer L, Chui H, et al. Head injury and the risk of AD in the MIRAGE study. Neurology. 2000;**54**(6):1316-1323

[93] Lee YK, Hou SW, Lee CC, Hsu CY, Huang YS, Su YC. Increased risk of dementia in patients with mild traumatic brain injury: A nationwide cohort study. PLoS One. 2013;**8**(5):e62422

[94] Smith DH, Chen XH, Pierce JE, Wolf JA, Trojanowski JQ, Graham DI, et al. Progressive atrophy and neuron death for one year following brain trauma in the rat. Journal of Neurotrauma. 1997;**14**(10):715-727

[95] Hong YT, Veenith T, Dewar D, Outtrim JG, Mani V, Williams C, et al. Amyloid imaging with carbon 11–Labeled Pittsburgh compound B for traumatic brain injury. JAMA Neurology. 2014;**71**(1):23-31

[96] Collins-Praino LE, Corrigan F. Does neuroinflammation drive the relationship between tau hyperphosphorylation and dementia development following traumatic brain injury? Brain, Behavior, and Immunity. 2017;**60**:369-382

[97] Lee CY, Landreth GE. The role of microglia in amyloid clearance from the AD brain. Journal of Neural Transmission (Vienna). 2010;**117**(8):949-960

[98] Sy M, Kitazawa M, Medeiros R, Whitman L, Cheng D, Lane TE, et al. Inflammation induced by infection potentiates tau pathological features in transgenic mice. The American Journal of Pathology. 2011;**178**(6):2811-2822

[99] Sheng JG, Zhu SG, Jones RA, Griffin WS, Mrak RE. Interleukin-1 promotes expression and phosphorylation of neurofilament and tau proteins in vivo. Experimental Neurology. 2000;**163**(2):388-391

[100] Bhaskar K, Konerth M, Kokiko-Cochran ON, Cardona A, Ransohoff RM, Lamb BT. Regulation of tau pathology by the microglial fractalkine receptor. Neuron. 2010;**68**(1):19-31

[101] Yoshiyama Y, Higuchi M, Zhang B, Huang SM, Iwata N, Saido TC, et al. Synapse loss and microglial activation precede tangles in a P301S tauopathy mouse model. Neuron. 2007;**53**(3):337-351

[102] Shi J-Q, Shen W, Chen J, Wang B-R, Zhong L-L, Zhu Y-W, et al. Anti-TNF-α reduces amyloid plaques and tau phosphorylation and induces CD11c-positive dendritic-like cell in the APP/PS1 transgenic mouse brains. Brain Research. 2011;**1368**:239-247

[103] Hull M, Eistetter J, Fiebich BL, Bauer J. Glutamate but not interleukin-6 influences the phosphorylation of tau in primary rat hippocampal neurons. Neuroscience Letters. 1999;**261**(1-2):33-36

[104] Li Y, Liu L, Barger SW, Griffin WS. Interleukin-1 mediates pathological effects of microglia on tau phosphorylation and on synaptophysin synthesis in cortical neurons through a p38-MAPK pathway. The Journal of Neuroscience. 2003;**23**(5):1605-1611

[105] Acosta SA, Tajiri N, Idl P, Bastawrous M, Sanberg PR, Kaneko Y, et al. Alpha-synuclein as a pathological link between chronic traumatic brain injury and Parkinson's disease. Journal of Cellular Physiology. 2015;**230**(5):1024-1032

[106] Saing T, Dick M, Nelson PT, Kim RC, Cribbs DH, Head E. Frontal cortex neuropathology in dementia pugilistica. Journal of Neurotrauma. 2012;**29**(6):1054-1070

[107] VanItallie TB. Traumatic brain injury (TBI) in collision sports: Possible mechanisms of transformation into chronic traumatic encephalopathy (CTE). Metabolism: Clinical and Experimental. 2019;**100S**:153943

[108] Cherry JD, Tripodis Y, Alvarez VE, Huber B, Kiernan PT, Daneshvar DH, et al. Microglial neuroinflammation contributes to tau accumulation in chronic traumatic encephalopathy. Acta Neuropathologica Communications. 2016;**4**(1):112

[109] Chancellor KB, Chancellor SE, Duke-Cohan JE, Huber BR, Stein TD, Alvarez VE, et al. Altered oligodendroglia and astroglia in chronic traumatic encephalopathy. Acta Neuropathologica. 2021;**142**(2):295-321

[110] Goldstein LE, Fisher AM, Tagge CA, Zhang XL, Velisek L, Sullivan JA, et al. Chronic traumatic encephalopathy in blast-exposed military veterans and a blast neurotrauma mouse model. Science Translational Medicine. 2012;**4**(134):134ra60

[111] McKee AC, Gavett BE, Stern RA, Nowinski CJ, Cantu RC, Kowall NW, et al. TDP-43 proteinopathy and motor neuron disease in chronic traumatic encephalopathy. Journal of Neuropathology and Experimental Neurology. 2010;**69**(9):918-929

[112] Falk D, Gibson KR. Evolutionary Anatomy of the Primate Cerebral Cortex. Cambridge: Cambridge University Press; 2001

[113] Xiong Y, Mahmood A, Chopp M. Animal models of traumatic brain injury. Nature Reviews Neuroscience. 2013;**14**(2):128

[114] Ho J, Kleiven S. Can sulci protect the brain from traumatic injury? Journal of Biomechanics. 2009;**42**(13):2074-2080

[115] Kinder HA, Baker EW, West FD. The pig as a preclinical traumatic brain injury model: Current models, functional outcome measures, and translational detection strategies. Neural Regeneration Research. 2019;**14**(3):413-424

[116] Ahmad AS, Satriotomo I, Fazal J, Nadeau SE, Dore S. Considerations for the optimization of induced white matter injury preclinical models. Frontiers in Neurology. 2015;**6**:172

[117] Dean DD, Frank JA, Turtzo LC. Controlled cortical impact in the rat. Current Protocols in Neuroscience. 2017;**81**:9.62.1-9.62.12

[118] Ma X, Aravind A, Pfister BJ, Chandra N, Haorah J. Animal models of traumatic brain injury and assessment of injury severity. Molecular Neurobiology. 2019;**56**(8):5332-5345

[119] Aravind A, Ravula AR, Chandra N, Pfister BJ. Behavioral deficits in animal models of blast traumatic brain injury. Frontiers in Neurology. 2020;**11**:990

[120] Ramilo O, Sáez-Llorens X, Mertsola J, Jafari H, Olsen KD, Hansen EJ, et al. Tumor necrosis factor alpha/ cachectin and interleukin 1 beta initiate meningeal inflammation. The Journal of Experimental Medicine. 1990;**172**(2):497-507

[121] Ross SA, Halliday MI, Campbell GC, Byrnes DP, Rowlands BJ. The presence of tumour necrosis factor in CSF and plasma after severe head injury. British Journal of Neurosurgery. 1994;**8**(4):419-425

[122] Scherbel U, Raghupathi R, Nakamura M, Saatman KE, Trojanowski JQ, Neugebauer E, et al. Differential acute and chronic responses of tumor necrosis factor-deficient mice to experimental brain injury. Proceedings of the National Academy of Sciences of the United States of America. 1999;**96**(15):8721-8726

[123] Perez-Barcena J, Ibáñez J, Brell M, Crespí C, Frontera G, Llompart-Pou JA, et al. Lack of correlation among intracerebral cytokines, intracranial pressure, and brain tissue oxygenation in patients with traumatic brain injury and diffuse lesions. Critical Care Medicine. 2011;**39**(3):533-540

[124] Winter CD, Pringle AK, Clough GF, Church MK. Raised parenchymal interleukin-6 levels correlate with improved outcome after traumatic brain injury. Brain: A Journal of Neurology. 2004;**127**(Pt 2):315-320

[125] Chamoun R, Suki D, Gopinath SP, Goodman JC, Robertson C. Role of extracellular glutamate measured by cerebral microdialysis in severe traumatic brain injury. Journal of Neurosurgery. 2010;**113**(3):564-570

[126] Wang YT, Edison P. Tau imaging in neurodegenerative diseases using positron emission tomography. Current Neurology and Neuroscience Reports. 2019;**19**(7):45

[127] Donat CK, Scott G, Gentleman SM, Sastre M. Microglial activation in traumatic brain injury. Frontiers in Aging Neuroscience. 2017;**9**:208

[128] Banati RB, Myers R, Kreutzberg GW. PK ('peripheral benzodiazepine')--binding sites in the CNS indicate early and discrete brain lesions: Microautoradiographic detection of [3H]PK11195 binding to activated microglia. Journal of Neurocytology. 1997;**26**(2):77-82

[129] Guo Y, Zeng H, Gao C. The role of neutrophil extracellular traps in central nervous system diseases and prospects for clinical application. Oxidative Medicine and Cellular Longevity. 2021;**2021**:9931742

[130] Hoyte LC, Brooks KJ, Nagel S, Akhtar A, Chen R, Mardiguian S, et al. Molecular magnetic resonance imaging of acute vascular cell adhesion molecule-1 expression in a mouse model of cerebral ischemia. Journal of Cerebral Blood Flow and Metabolism. 2010;**30**(6):1178-1187

[131] McAteer MA, Sibson NR, von Zur MC, Schneider JE, Lowe AS, Warrick N, et al. In vivo magnetic resonance imaging of acute brain inflammation using microparticles of iron oxide. Nature Medicine. 2007;**13**(10):1253-1258

[132] Gauberti M, Montagne A, Marcos-Contreras OA, Le Behot A, Maubert E, Vivien D. Ultra-sensitive molecular MRI of vascular cell adhesion molecule-1 reveals a dynamic inflammatory penumbra after strokes. Stroke. 2013;**44**(7):1988-1996

[133] Ma Y, Liu Y, Ruan X, Liu X, Zheng J, Teng H, et al. Gene expression signature of traumatic brain injury. Frontiers in Genetics. 2021;**12**:646436

[134] Lynch JR, Wang H, Mace B, Leinenweber S, Warner DS, Bennett ER, et al. A novel therapeutic derived from apolipoprotein E reduces brain inflammation and improves outcome after closed head injury. Experimental Neurology. 2005;**192**(1):109-116

[135] Sowers JL, Wu P, Zhang K, DeWitt DS, Prough DS. Proteomic changes in traumatic brain injury: Experimental approaches. Current Opinion in Neurology. 2018;**31**(6):709-717

[136] Chen X, Chen C, Fan S, Wu S, Yang F, Fang Z, et al. Omega-3 polyunsaturated fatty acid attenuates the inflammatory response by modulating microglia polarization through SIRT1-mediated deacetylation of the HMGB1/NF-κB pathway following experimental traumatic brain injury. Journal of Neuroinflammation. 2018;**15**(1):116

[137] Roberts I, Yates D, Sandercock P, Farrell B, Wasserberg J, Lomas G, et al. Effect of intravenous corticosteroids on death within 14 days in 10008 adults with clinically significant head injury (MRC CRASH trial): Randomised placebo-controlled trial. Lancet. 2004;**364**(9442):1321-1328

[138] Girgis H, Palmier B, Croci N, Soustrat M, Plotkine M, Marchand-Leroux C. Effects of selective and non-selective cyclooxygenase inhibition against neurological deficit and brain oedema following closed head injury in mice. Brain Research. 2013;**1491**:78-87

[139] Wallenquist U, Holmqvist K, Hånell A, Marklund N, Hillered L, Forsberg-Nilsson K. Ibuprofen attenuates the inflammatory response and allows formation of migratory neuroblasts from grafted stem cells after traumatic brain injury. Restorative Neurology and Neuroscience. 2012;**30**(1):9-19

[140] Browne K, Iwata A, Putt M, Smith D. Chronic ibuprofen administration worsens cognitive

outcome following traumatic brain injury in rats. Experimental Neurology. 2006;**201**(2):301-307

[141] Parepally JMR, Mandula H, Smith QR. Brain uptake of nonsteroidal anti-inflammatory drugs: Ibuprofen, flurbiprofen, and indomethacin. Pharmaceutical Research. 2006;**23**(5):873-881

[142] Martín-Saborido C, López-Alcalde J, Ciapponi A, Sánchez Martín CE, Garcia Garcia E, Escobar Aguilar G, et al. Indomethacin for intracranial hypertension secondary to severe traumatic brain injury in adults. Cochrane Database of Systematic Reviews. 2019;**2019**(11):CD011725

[143] Bye N, Habgood MD, Callaway JK, Malakooti N, Potter A, Kossmann T, et al. Transient neuroprotection by minocycline following traumatic brain injury is associated with attenuated microglial activation but no changes in cell apoptosis or neutrophil infiltration. Experimental Neurology. 2007;**204**(1):220-233

[144] Homsi S, Federico F, Croci N, Palmier B, Plotkine M, Marchand-Leroux C, et al. Minocycline effects on cerebral edema: Relations with inflammatory and oxidative stress markers following traumatic brain injury in mice. Brain Research. 2009;**1291**:122-132

[145] Yrjänheikki J, Keinänen R, Pellikka M, Hökfelt T, Koistinaho J. Tetracyclines inhibit microglial activation and are neuroprotective in global brain ischemia. Proceedings of the National Academy of Sciences. 1998;**95**(26):15769-15774

[146] Meythaler J, Fath J, Fuerst D, Zokary H, Freese K, Martin HB, et al. Safety and feasibility of minocycline in treatment of acute traumatic brain injury. Brain Injury. 2019;**33**(5):679-689

[147] Gordon PH, Moore DH, Miller RG, Florence JM, Verheijde JL, Doorish C, et al. Efficacy of minocycline in patients with amyotrophic lateral sclerosis: A phase III randomised trial. The Lancet Neurology. 2007;**6**(12):1045-1053

[148] Bramlett HM, Dietrich WD. Long-term consequences of traumatic brain injury: Current status of potential mechanisms of injury and neurological outcomes. Journal of Neurotrauma. 2015;**32**(23):1834-1848

[149] Webster KM, Sun M, Crack P, O'Brien TJ, Shultz SR, Semple BD. Inflammation in epileptogenesis after traumatic brain injury. Journal of Neuroinflammation. 2017;**14**(1):10

[150] Kirmani BF, Robinson DM, Fonkem E, Graf K, Huang JH. Role of anticonvulsants in the management of posttraumatic epilepsy. Frontiers in Neurology. 2016;**7**:32

[151] Kim J-E, Choi H-C, Song H-K, Jo S-M, Kim D-S, Choi S-Y, et al. Levetiracetam inhibits interleukin-1β inflammatory responses in the hippocampus and piriform cortex of epileptic rats. Neuroscience Letters. 2010;**471**(2):94-99

[152] Dambach H, Hinkerohe D, Prochnow N, Stienen MN, Moinfar Z, Haase CG, et al. Glia and epilepsy: Experimental investigation of antiepileptic drugs in an astroglia/microglia co-culture model of inflammation. Epilepsia. 2014;**55**(1):184-192

[153] Schreibman DL, Hong CM, Keledjian K, Ivanova S, Tsymbalyuk S, Gerzanich V, et al. Mannitol and hypertonic saline reduce

swelling and modulate inflammatory markers in a rat model of intracerebral Hemorrhage. Neurocritical Care. 2018;**29**(2):253-263

[154] Rhind SG, Crnko NT, Baker AJ, Morrison LJ, Shek PN, Scarpelini S, et al. Prehospital resuscitation with hypertonic saline-dextran modulates inflammatory, coagulation and endothelial activation marker profiles in severe traumatic brain injured patients. Journal of Neuroinflammation. 2010;**7**(1):5

[155] Zeng HK, Wang QS, Deng YY, Fang M, Chen CB, Fu YH, et al. Hypertonic saline ameliorates cerebral edema through downregulation of aquaporin-4 expression in the astrocytes. Neuroscience. 2010;**166**(3):878-885

[156] Roquilly A, Moyer JD, Huet O, Lasocki S, Cohen B, Dahyot-Fizelier C, et al. Effect of continuous infusion of hypertonic saline vs standard care on 6-month neurological outcomes in patients with traumatic brain injury. Journal of the American Medical Association. 2021;**325**(20):2056

[157] Collaborators C-t. Effects of tranexamic acid on death, disability, vascular occlusive events and other morbidities in patients with acute traumatic brain injury (CRASH-3): A randomised, placebo-controlled trial. Lancet. 2019;**394**(10210):1713-1723

[158] Barrett CD, Moore HB, Kong Y-W, Chapman MP, Sriram G, Lim D, et al. Tranexamic acid mediates proinflammatory and anti-inflammatory signaling via complement C5a regulation in a plasminogen activator–dependent manner. Journal of Trauma and Acute Care Surgery. 2019;**86**(1):101-107

[159] Grant AL, Letson HL, Morris JL, McEwen P, Hazratwala K, Wilkinson M, et al. Tranexamic acid is associated with selective increase in inflammatory markers following total knee arthroplasty (TKA): A pilot study. Journal of Orthopaedic Surgery and Research. 2018;**13**(1):149

[160] Wu X, Benov A, Darlington DN, Keesee JD, Liu B, Cap AP. Effect of tranexamic acid administration on acute traumatic coagulopathy in rats with polytrauma and hemorrhage. PLoS One. 2019;**14**(10):e0223406-e

[161] Boudreau RM, Johnson M, Veile R, Friend LA, Goetzman H, Pritts TA, et al. Impact of tranexamic acid on coagulation and inflammation in murine models of traumatic brain injury and hemorrhage. Journal of Surgical Research. 2017;**215**: 47-54

[162] Lotocki G, de Rivero Vaccari JP, Perez ER, Alonso OF, Curbelo K, Keane RW, et al. Therapeutic hypothermia modulates TNFR1 signaling in the traumatized brain via early transient activation of the JNK pathway and suppression of XIAP cleavage. European Journal of Neuroscience. 2006;**24**(8):2283-2290

[163] Crossley S, Reid J, McLatchie R, Hayton J, Clark C, MacDougall M, et al. A systematic review of therapeutic hypothermia for adult patients following traumatic brain injury. Critical Care. 2014;**18**(2):R75-R7R

[164] Timaru-Kast R, Luh C, Gotthardt P, Huang C, Schafer MK, Engelhard K, et al. Influence of age on brain edema formation, secondary brain damage and inflammatory response after brain trauma in mice. PLoS One. 2012;**7**(8):e43829

[165] Morganti JM, Riparip LK, Chou A, Liu S, Gupta N, Rosi S. Age exacerbates the CCR2/5-mediated

neuroinflammatory response to traumatic brain injury. Journal of Neuroinflammation. 2016;**13**(1):80

[166] Delage C, Taib T, Mamma C, Lerouet D, Besson VC. Traumatic brain injury: An age-dependent view of post-traumatic neuroinflammation and its treatment. Pharmaceutics. 2021;**13**(10)

[167] Appelberg KS, Hovda DA, Prins ML. The effects of a ketogenic diet on behavioral outcome after controlled cortical impact injury in the juvenile and adult rat. Journal of Neurotrauma. 2009;**26**(4):497-506

[168] Prins ML, Fujima LS, Hovda DA. Age-dependent reduction of cortical contusion volume by ketones after traumatic brain injury. Journal of Neuroscience Research. 2005;**82**(3):413-420

[169] Djebaili M, Hoffman SW, Stein DG. Allopregnanolone and progesterone decrease cell death and cognitive deficits after a contusion of the rat pre-frontal cortex. Neuroscience. 2004;**123**(2):349-359

[170] Barreto G, Veiga S, Azcoitia I, Garcia-Segura LM, Garcia-Ovejero D. Testosterone decreases reactive astroglia and reactive microglia after brain injury in male rats: Role of its metabolites, oestradiol and dihydrotestosterone. The European Journal of Neuroscience. 2007;**25**(10):3039-3046

[171] Ma C, Wu X, Shen X, Yang Y, Chen Z, Sun X, et al. Sex differences in traumatic brain injury: A multi-dimensional exploration in genes, hormones, cells, individuals, and society. Chinese Neurosurgical Journal. 2019;**5**:24

[172] Bergold PJ. Treatment of traumatic brain injury with anti-inflammatory drugs. Experimental Neurology. 2016;**275**(Pt 3):367-380

[173] Garrett MC, Otten ML, Starke RM, Komotar RJ, Magotti P, Lambris JD, et al. Synergistic neuroprotective effects of C3a and C5a receptor blockade following intracerebral hemorrhage. Brain Research. 2009;**1298**:171-177

[174] Imam AM, Jin G, Duggan M, Sillesen M, Hwabejire JO, Jepsen CH, et al. Synergistic effects of fresh frozen plasma and valproic acid treatment in a combined model of traumatic brain injury and hemorrhagic shock. Surgery. 2013;**154**(2):388-396

[175] Tang H, Hua F, Wang J, Yousuf S, Atif F, Sayeed I, et al. Progesterone and vitamin D combination therapy modulates inflammatory response after traumatic brain injury. Brain Injury. 2015;**29**(10):1165-1174

[176] Abu Hamdeh S, Tenovuo O, Peul W, Marklund N. "Omics" in traumatic brain injury: Novel approaches to a complex disease. Acta Neurochirurgica. 2021;**163**(9):2581-2594

[177] Lurie DI. An integrative approach to neuroinflammation in psychiatric disorders and neuropathic pain. Journal of Experimental Neuroscience. 2018;**12**:1179069518793639

[178] Shaito A, Hasan H, Habashy KJ, Fakih W, Abdelhady S, Ahmad F, et al. Western diet aggravates neuronal insult in post-traumatic brain injury: Proposed pathways for interplay. eBioMedicine. 2020;**57**:102829

[179] Yu J, Zhu H, Taheri S, Mondy W, Perry S, Kindy MS. Impact of nutrition on inflammation, tauopathy, and behavioral outcomes from chronic traumatic encephalopathy. Journal of Neuroinflammation. 2018;**15**(1):277

Section 2

Specialties

Chapter 4

Penetrating Craniocerebral Injury in Pediatric Patients

Jillian Plonsker, Michael Brandel, Usman Khan and Michael L. Levy

Abstract

Penetrating head trauma is rare in the pediatric population, and rarer still in the civilian pediatric population. The high rehabilitation potential of children and the higher likelihood of a low-velocity, survivable injury necessitates careful management to minimize morbidity due to secondary injury from ischemia or infection. Management of penetrating injuries includes patient stabilization, appropriate imaging, and if surgery is needed, entry/exit site debridement with dural closure to prevent cerebrospinal fluid leak. Post-operative care includes infection prevention, intracerebral pressure management, and early identification of vasospasm and pseudoaneurysm formation.

Keywords: pediatric, penetrating head injury, low-velocity, non-missile, vasospasm, pseudoaneurysm

1. Introduction

Although rare, penetrating craniocerebral injury is an increasingly recognized cause of emergent neurosurgical admissions in children and adolescents 17 years of age or younger [1]. Outside of war zones, these injuries can occur in the setting of gang-related violence in major metropolitan areas. Penetrating head injury may result from gunshot wounds or stabbings, and less commonly due to non-powder guns (Zip Guns) or transorbital penetration [2, 3]. In this review, we have defined high-velocity injuries as those that result from projectiles/objects traveling at velocities >600 meters per second. These are most commonly the result of rifle injuries, which are more prevalent in military conflicts. Low-velocity injuries are usually the result of handguns in civilian populations. The low-velocity equivalents in military conflicts include both handgun and shrapnel injuries. Additional low-velocity mechanisms of injury in children can include BB and pellet gun injuries, stab injuries, blunt penetrating injury, and trauma resulting from pencils, branches, nails, and other objects.

A relatively small number of case series in varied settings comprise the majority of the pediatric literature on penetrating craniocerebral injury.

Barlow et al. study of gunshot wounds in 108 children (nine cerebral injuries) at Harlem Hospital over 10 years was among the first series to examine the demographic, intentionality, and cause of these types of injuries in children [4].

Most worrisome was that 53% of the guns belonged to the children themselves, and 8% of injuries were inflicted by the police.

Beaver et al. reviewed 132 children under 16 years with fatal firearm injuries in the state of Maryland [5]. The cause of death was a homicide in 46%, accident in 25%, and suicide in 22%. Deaths occurred at home in 75% of cases. The perpetrator was a friend in 21%, family member in 20%, acquaintance in 7%, a bystander in 2%, and self-inflicted in 30%.

In 1993, Levy et al. published their experience with 105 pediatric patients at the University of Southern California/Los Angeles County Medical Center with a diagnosis of a gunshot wound to the brain during an 8-year period [1]. Most of these injuries (72%) were gang-related or secondary to murder-suicide, in contrast to a much higher rate of suicide in the adult population. These findings were contextualized by rising rates of gang-related murders in Los Angeles County and increasing numbers of gang members in that time frame. Similarly, a prior study by Ordog et al. [6] described 34 patients, 10 years of age or younger who were treated for gunshot wounds in Los Angeles between 1980 and 1987, noting that no children in this age range had been treated for gunshot wounds prior to 1980.

A retrospective review of traumatic injuries in children 16 years or younger in the San Francisco bay area from 2000 to 2009 revealed that the incidence of gunshot wounds to the head in children continued to increase over time. This represents another study documenting the vexatious number of these injuries each year in children [7]. These injuries were associated with a 63% mortality rate and were thought to represent mostly intentional injuries.

Bandt et al. reported their experience with 48 patients less than 18 years of age with penetrating intracranial gunshot injuries between 2002 and 2011 in St. Louis, MO [8]. The authors proposed a management paradigm involving more aggressive treatment compared to adults due to the more favorable outcomes experienced by children.

Seventy-one pediatric patients with an intracranial gunshot wound between 1996 and 2013 in Memphis, TN were analyzed by Decuypere et al. [9]. Nearly half of the victims died from their injuries, but over 80% of survivors had a good outcome. As noted in prior studies, the authors reported that variables related to the initial clinical exam and classification of CT findings were found to be the most important predictors of outcome.

Thirty patients under the age of 13 years who suffered craniocerebral gunshot injuries were treated at Red Cross War Memorial Children's Hospital in South Africa between 1989 and 2001 [10]. Over half of the victims were injured in the crossfire of civilian violence.

A case series from Mashhad, Iran reported 14 penetrating head injuries in children less than 10 years [11]. These injuries were primarily due to low-velocity objects, such as pencils, rods, silverware, and other miscellaneous objects. The authors noted that pediatric civilian low-velocity gunshot injuries were comparatively uncommon in some middle eastern countries and Japan as compared to the United States and Europe. These findings have supported the prior literature which documented the significant number of gunshot-related injuries to the head in the United States as compared to other countries.

A series from Tel Aviv concluded that pediatric craniocerebral gunshot injuries from plastic projectiles resembled those of low-velocity missiles, with similar treatment algorithms and outcomes compared to other penetrating craniocerebral injuries in civilians [12].

Low-velocity penetrating injuries in children are not as common in armed conflict. Given the nature of the high-velocity injuries associated with rifles, most low-velocity injuries are the result of penetrating shrapnel. Low-velocity injuries are those associated with projectiles traveling less than 600 m/sec. This is consistent with the prevalence of handgun injuries in civilian populations. Wani et al. reported on 51 children with penetrating brain injuries who were the victims of armed conflict [13]. Nearly all injuries were from roadside grenade attacks. Victims of grenade attacks had better outcomes than those who suffered bullet injuries to the head. The authors noted that being upright and running away from an audible attack may have predisposed patients to craniocerebral injury, which perhaps could have been prevented by lying down.

A large series of cranial stab wounds was published by Domingo et al. in 1994, including 54 patients less than 14 years. Injuries were due to assault in 58% and accidental in 42%. All patients survived their injury and required surgical debridement [14]. A large series on pediatric penetrating brain injury in Durban, South Africa included more stab wounds (57%) than gunshot wounds (43%) [15]. Interestingly, neurological deficits did not significantly differ by the mechanism of injury when accounting for age and other clinical information.

Irfan et al. reported their experience with four patients in the 2–3 year age range who experienced gunshot wounds to the head, only one of whom did not survive [16]. Penetrating craniocerebral injuries to patients in this age range have the additional nuance of developmental and neurobehavioral impact among survivors [17].

2. Epidemiology

Due to the rarity of penetrating craniocerebral injury in children, it is challenging to identify epidemiological data. This is particularly true given the diversity of data sources reported in the aforementioned case series.

The incidence of pediatric TBI ranges from 12 to 700 per 100,000 population, with most studies reporting between 47 and 280 [18–20]. While the incidence of penetrating TBI in children remains unknown, it represents a small fraction of those likely between 1% and 7%, and varies significantly by country and setting [15, 21].

An analysis of the National Trauma Data Bank, a curated United States trauma registry, demonstrated that gunshot wounds to the head represented 1.4% of pediatric TBI cases, with increasing incidence over time (from 275 per 100,000 in 2003 to 315 per 100,000 in 2012). The mean age was 14.8 years and 79.2% were male. Most victims were African American (43%) or white (35%). Assault was the most common mechanism (63%), followed by suicide (18.3%) and accident (12.6%). There was a time trend for increasing suicides, decreasing accidental injuries, and a stable assault rate. The location of injury was commonly residential (40.6%) or street (24.9%), and less often a public building (1.9%) or recreational location (0.9%). Mortality was 45.1% overall, and 71.5% in the setting of suicidal intent.

In general, pediatric gunshot wound victims were primarily males with mortality rates ranging from 47.9–65% [1, 6, 8–10, 15, 22–25].

Among TBI patients, children in racial minority groups or of low-income status are more likely to be the victim of assault or firearms and are more likely to have poor clinical outcomes [26]. This is likely also true, specifically, for victims of penetrating TBI [21], although data are limited.

3. Management

Initial management of both high- and low-velocity penetrating injury in children involves emergent and aggressive hemodynamic stabilization, correction of coagulopathies, and neurologic assessment. Neurologic imaging after stabilization should include brain computed topography (CT) [27]. CT angiography should be considered to rule out vascular injury. An intracranial pressure monitor is indicated in patients with a low Glasgow coma score (GCS) ≤ 7 or signs of elevated intracranial pressure.

The rate of surgical intervention ranges from 51 to 100% for injuries due to gunshot wounds or explosives [9, 10, 22–24], 70–94% in pellet gun injuries [28, 29], 60% in dog bites [30], and up to100% in stab wounds [14]. Lower rates of intervention among high-velocity injuries likely reflect nonsurvivors or those with inoperable injuries.

Goals of surgery depend on the extent of the injury [31]. Small head wounds without significant intracranial pathology may simply require local wound care and closure, whereas devitalized scalp or compromised bone and dura may require more extensive debridement. Intracranial injuries with hematomas and/or mass effect may require debridement of necrotic brain tissue and accessible bone fragments, or hematoma evacuation. Debridement of the missile tract and the aggressive pursuit of bone/metallic fragments is not recommended when there is no significant mass effect (**Figure 1**). As noted in adult populations a primary goal of surgical intervention in children is dural closure to avoid CSF leaks. Antiepileptic and antimicrobial recommendations are discussed in the following section.

4. Complications

4.1 Structural

Direct impact from the penetrating object can cause a variety of damage to tissue. Skull fracture and cerebrospinal fluid leak due to dural laceration are common. Children's skulls do not become fully ossified until two years of age; therefore, they are more susceptible to skull fracture after non-missile or low-velocity penetrating trauma. The most common entry locations are the thin-walled orbit and the squamous temporal bone [32–34]. Bihemispheric injury and ventricular transgression are associated with worse outcomes (**Figure 2**).

Low-velocity objects are, however, less likely to cause contra-coup injuries, thermal or blast injuries than are high-velocity or missile objects [34]. Depending on the course of the object through brain tissue, there may be a hematoma or cerebral contusion causing a mass effect.

4.2 Neurologic

The significance of the trajectory of the object/projectile is that it has been found to be a powerful determinant of outcome (both morbidity and mortality) as previously noted. The trajectory of the object impacts the likelihood of a transient or permanent neurologic deficit, which most commonly are weakness and cranial

DOI: http://dx.doi.org/10.5772/intechopen.106549

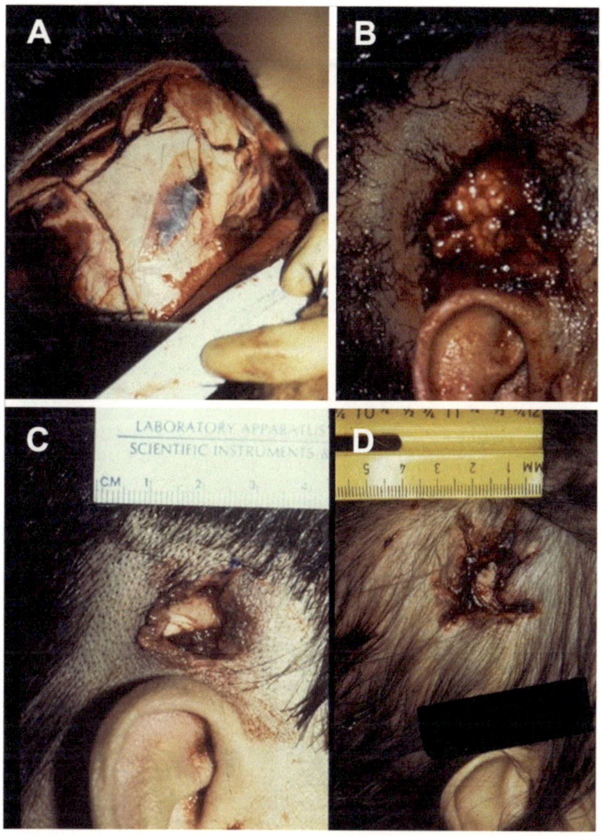

Figure 1.
A–D. Entry wound and exit wound should be debrided in the operating room with removal of superficial foreign material and repair of any dural injury.

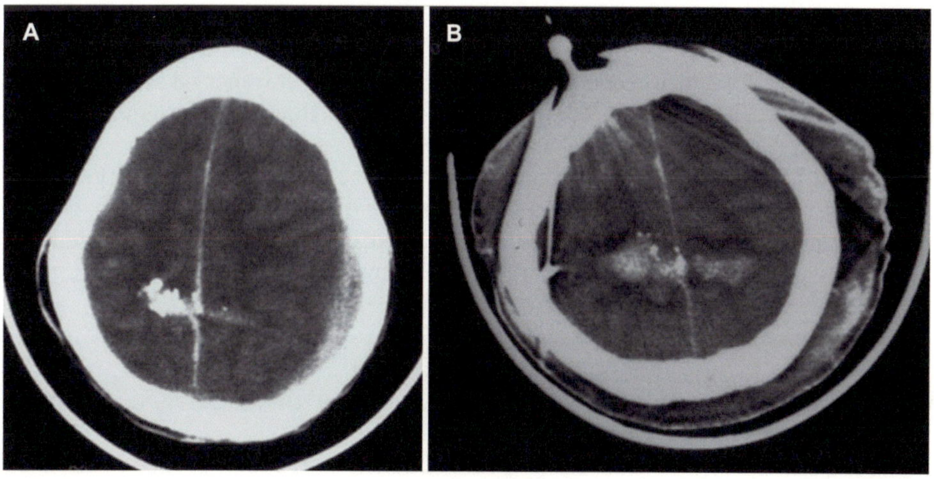

Figure 2.
A–B. Bihemispheric injury is associated with a worse prognosis.

neuropathy. A review of 223 patients with a near-even mix of high and low-velocity injury found that the mean age of children with the neurologic deficit was higher (11.72 years) than those who were neurologically intact (8.96 years) [15].

The routine use of antiepileptics is controversial. Trauma literature supports the use of antiepileptics for the prevention of early (<7 days) post-traumatic epilepsy but not late post-traumatic epilepsy [34, 35]. Low GCS is independently associated with developing post-traumatic seizures in pediatric patients [36]. Left-sided injury is also reported to be associated with a higher likelihood of seizures [15].

Newer antiepileptics, such as levetiracetam, have not been as rigorously studied for use in this patient population despite their popularity. Additionally, there is a disparity in pediatric literature compared to adult literature regarding the routine use of antiepileptics after traumatic brain injury. It seems to be routine practice in moderate to severe penetrating head trauma to administer prophylactic antiepileptics due to the low-risk profile, though this remains at the discretion of the treating neurosurgeon and there is not enough literature support to define management standards.

Blunt traumatic brain injury has been associated with a high rate of new diagnoses of ADHD, oppositional defiant disorder, mood disorders, PTSD, OCD, bipolar disorder, and antisocial or aggressive behaviors. Although perhaps of less importance in the acute period, penetrating head trauma, particularly to the frontal lobe, may cause devastating neuropsychiatric sequelae in children. Neuropsychiatric evaluation and referral to child psychiatry should always be considered [37].

4.3 Infectious

The routine use of broad-spectrum empiric antibiotics after penetrating head trauma is common but not universally agreed upon. Complications of grossly contaminated wounds include cerebritis, intracerebral abscess, ventriculitis, and meningitis. The most common pathogens are *Staphylococcus* species and gram-negative bacteria, though anaerobic species have been reported in both pediatric and adult cases with high mortality [34, 38]. Empiric antibiotic therapy should cover for these most common pathogens. There is considerable variability in the literature as to the exact type of antibiotics and the length of therapy. Early surgical intervention and debridement <12 hours from presentation decrease the risk of subsequent infection, with watertight dural closure being one of the most significant variables related to minimizing infection [34, 39].

Pediatric series of penetrating head trauma report a higher rate of infection than adults, up to 40–50% [40]. Risk factors for infection include the foreign body being a porous material, such as wood, fragmentation of the object, cerebrospinal fluid leak, nasal or mastoid sinus involvement, and gross contamination of the entry or exit site (**Figure 3**).

Low-velocity penetrating injuries, which are more common in young patients, are more likely to be grossly contaminated with skin, hair, and bone along the projectile tract. They are also more likely to involve porous material that can fragment, further increasing the risk of infection.

While most studies recommend immediate initiation of broad-spectrum antibiotics on arrival to the emergency department, a large retrospective review of adult trauma patients in Cleveland, OH described a very low incidence of infection despite most patients only receiving one dose of Ancef [39].

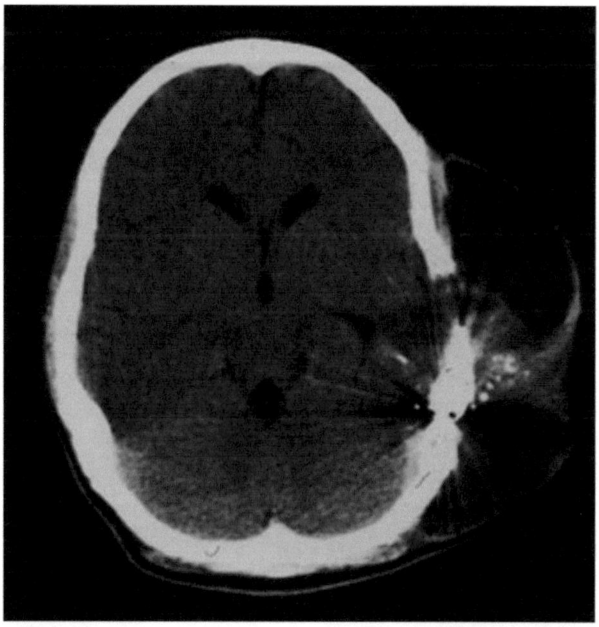

Figure 3.
Dural laceration and the cerebrospinal fluid leak should be addressed urgently in the operating room to reduce the likelihood of infection.

4.4 Vascular

Morbidity after penetrating head trauma can be significantly impacted by both immediate and delayed vascular pathology. Immediate injury to the vasculature or direct tissue injury can lead to significant blood loss, space-occupying hematoma, or cerebral ischemia, all of which may cause neurologic deficit or secondary injury due to cerebral edema and elevated intracranial pressure [41].

Traumatic intracranial pseudoaneurysms are a relatively common sequelae of both blunt and penetrating head trauma; 20% of traumatic aneurysms are related to penetrating head trauma. The most common vessels involved are the MCA, followed by the ACA and the ICA [Alvis]. The rupture risk of traumatic pseudoaneurysms resultant from penetrating injury is not well quantified, and they may grow or shrink with time. However, the presence of subarachnoid hemorrhage after penetrating head trauma has been significantly associated with mortality (**Figure 4**). At 48 hours post-injury, 17% of survivors and 68% of nonsurvivors had SAH on imaging [42]. Vascular imaging should be strongly considered for any penetrating trauma in which the object tract traverses the Sylvian fissure or any major subarachnoid space or is adjacent to vascular structures. CTA is rapid and convenient, however, may be obscured by an artifact of metallic objects and, therefore, formal angiography might be necessary. Aneurysms can form in the days following trauma or may form in a delayed fashion. Surgical or interventional treatment is recommended due to the high risk of rupture [43, 44].

Vasospasm after penetrating pediatric head trauma may be an underrecognized phenomenon contributing to preventable "secondary" brain injury by reducing cerebral perfusion. A prospective study of pediatric patients with blunt traumatic brain

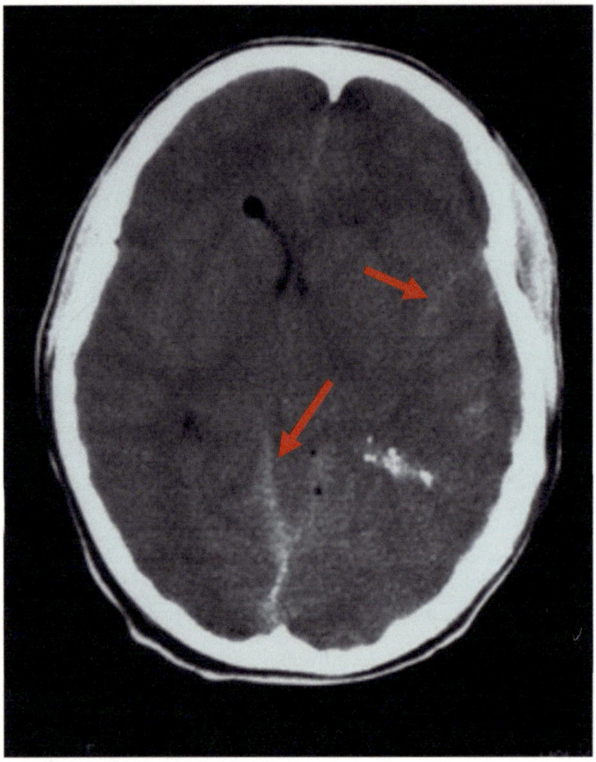

Figure 4.
Subarachnoid hemorrhage is a significant predictor of mortality.

injury demonstrated a moderately high prevalence of vasospasm on transcranial doppler (TCD), which was correlated with the severity of the injury. This study further identified post-resuscitation GCS < 8, mechanism of injury (motor vehicle accident), and fever at admission as significant predictors of subsequent development of vasospasm [45]. In adults with penetrating trauma, the incidence of vasospasm is as high as 40% and has a strong association with the presence of subarachnoid hemorrhage [46]. Vasospasm occurs in 21% of blunt moderate to severe TBI patients, and 33.5% of severe TBI patients studied with TCD. Peak onset is 2–4 days post-injury and resolves in 2–3 days [45]. Vasospasm following low-velocity penetrating trauma has also been described. Given that these injuries are less likely to be lethal and have the potential for a good outcome, prevention of secondary injury is paramount [47].

The anticipation and presumptive treatment to avoid concomitant infection are essential. Associated cerebritis, abscess, or sepsis can be additionally associated with stroke. This is an important consideration in an immunocompromised patient. Additionally, stroke-associated pneumonia (SAP) can increase morbidity and mortality following these injuries.

5. Conclusions

Pediatric penetrating head trauma in civilian populations is rare. Children in these settings are more likely to be struck by low-velocity or non-missile objects than by firearms, which confer a higher likelihood of survival. Therefore, surgical debridement or decompression, closure of dural violations to prevent infection, and diligent medical management to prevent secondary injury are critical to maximizing recovery in this resilient patient population.

Author details

Jillian Plonsker[1], Michael Brandel[1], Usman Khan[1] and Michael L. Levy[1,2*]

1 Department of Neurological Surgery, University of California San Diego Health, La Jolla, CA, USA

2 Pediatric Neurosurgery Division, Rady Children's Hospital, San Diego, CA, USA

*Address all correspondence to: mlevy@rchsd.org

References

[1] Levy ML et al. Penetrating craniocerebral injury resultant from gunshot wounds: Gang-related injury in children and adolescents. Neurosurgery. 1993;**33**(6):1018-1024 discussion 1024-5

[2] Santiago-Dieppa DR et al. BB gunshot wound to the head. The Journal of Pediatrics. 2019;**210**:237

[3] Di Roio C et al. Craniocerebral injury resulting from transorbital stick penetration in children. Child's Nervous System. 2000;**16**(8):503-506 discussion 507

[4] Barlow B, Niemirska M, Gandhi RP. Ten years' experience with pediatric gunshot wounds. Journal of Pediatric Surgery. 1982;**17**(6):927-932

[5] Beaver BL et al. Characteristics of pediatric firearm fatalities. Journal of Pediatric Surgery. 1990;**25**(1):97-99 discussion 99-100

[6] Ordog GJ et al. Gunshot wounds in children under 10 years of age. A new epidemic. American Journal of Diseases of Children. 1988;**142**(6):618-622

[7] Schecter SC et al. Pediatric penetrating trauma: The epidemic continues. Journal of Trauma and Acute Care Surgery. 2012;**73**(3):721-725

[8] Bandt SK et al. Management of pediatric intracranial gunshot wounds: Predictors of favorable clinical outcome and a new proposed treatment paradigm. Journal of Neurosurgery. Pediatrics. 2012;**10**(6):511-517

[9] DeCuypere M et al. Pediatric intracranial gunshot wounds: The Memphis experience. Journal of Neurosurgery. Pediatrics. 2016;**17**(5):595-601

[10] Coughlan MD et al. Craniocerebral gunshot injuries in children. Child's Nervous System. 2003;**19**(5-6):348-352

[11] Faraji M, Ashrafzadeh F. Penetrating head injuries in children. Neurosurgery Quarterly. 2005;**15**(3):160-163

[12] Paret G et al. Pediatric craniocerebral wounds from plastic bullets: Prognostic implications, course, and outcome. The Journal of Trauma. 1996;**41**(5):859-863

[13] Wani AA et al. Missile injury to the pediatric brain in conflict zones. Journal of Neurosurgery. Pediatrics. 2011;**7**(3):276-281

[14] Domingo Z, Peter JC, de Villiers JC. Low-velocity penetrating craniocerebral injury in childhood. Pediatric Neurosurgery. 1994;**21**(1):45-49

[15] Muballe KD, Hardcastle T, Kiratu E. Neurological findings in pediatric penetrating head injury at a university teaching hospital in Durban, South Africa: A 23-year retrospective study. Journal of Neurosurgery. Pediatrics. 2016;**18**(5):550-557

[16] Irfan FB et al. Craniocerebral gunshot injuries in preschoolers. Child's Nervous System. 2010;**26**(1):61-66

[17] Ewing-Cobbs L et al. Gunshot wounds to the brain in children and adolescents: Age and neurobehavioral development. Neurosurgery. 1994;**35**(2):225-233 discussion 233

[18] Mikhael M, Frost E, Cristancho M. Perioperative Care for Pediatric Patients with Penetrating Brain Injury: A review.

Journal of Neurosurgical Anesthesiology. 2018;**30**(4):290-298

[19] Dewan MC et al. Epidemiology of global Pediatric traumatic brain injury: Qualitative review. World Neurosurgery. 2016;**91**:497-509.e1

[20] Thurman DJ. The epidemiology of traumatic brain injury in children and youths: A review of research since 1990. Journal of Child Neurology. 2016;**31**(1):20-27

[21] Hansen D, Yue JK, Winkler EA, Dhall SS, Manley GT, Tarapore PE. Pediatric firearm-related traumatic brain injury in United States trauma centers. Journal of Neurosurgery: Pediatrics PED. 2019;**24**(5):498-508

[22] Klimo P et al. Severe Pediatric head injury during the Iraq and Afghanistan conflicts. Neurosurgery. 2015;**77**(1):1-7 discussion 7

[23] Mathew P et al. Operative treatment of paediatric penetrating head injuries in southern Afghanistan. British Journal of Neurosurgery. 2013;**27**(4):489-496

[24] Paret G et al. Gunshot wounds in brains of children: Prognostic variables in mortality, course, and outcome. Journal of Neurotrauma. 1998;**15**(11):967-972

[25] Miner ME et al. The results of treatment of gunshot wounds to the brain in children. Neurosurgery. 1990;**26**(1):20-24 discussion 24-5

[26] Kelly KA, Patel PD, Salwi S, Lovvorn HN III, Naftel R. Socioeconomic health disparities in pediatric traumatic brain injury on a national level. Journal of Neurosurgery: Pediatrics. 2022;**29**(3):335-341

[27] Alvis-Miranda HR et al. Craniocerebral gunshot injuries; a review of the current literature. Bulletin of Emergency and Trauma. 2016;**4**(2):65-74

[28] Kumar R et al. Penetrating head injuries in children due to BB and pellet guns: A poorly recognized public health risk. Journal of Neurosurgery. Pediatrics. 2016;**17**(2):215-221

[29] Amirjamshidi A, Abbassioun K, Roosbeh H. Air-gun pellet injuries to the head and neck. Surgical Neurology. 1997;**47**(4):331-338

[30] Steen T et al. Intracranial injuries from dog bites in children. Pediatric Neurosurgery. 2015;**50**(4):187-195

[31] Surgical Management of Penetrating Brain Injury. The Journal of Trauma: Injury, Infection, and Critical Care. 2001;**51**(2):S16-S25

[32] Torche VE, Rojas VP, Vera FF, Vigueras A. Lesión penetrante intracraneana transorbitaria, con compromiso de seno cavernoso en paciente pediátrico. Neurocirugia. 2021

[33] Varutti R, Mosca A, Latronico N. Non-visible penetrating brain trauma: A case report. Journal of Emergency Practice and Trauma. 2020;**6**(1):50-52

[34] Drosos E et al. Pediatric nonmissile penetrating head injury: Case series and literature review. World Neurosurgery. 2018;**110**:193-205

[35] Aarabi B et al. Antiseizure prophylaxis for penetrating brain injury (vol 51, pg S41, 2001). Journal of Trauma and Acute Care Surgery. 2017;**83**(6):1218-1218

[36] Lewis RJ et al. Clinical predictors of post-traumatic seizures in children with head trauma. Annals of Emergency Medicine. 1993;**22**(7):1114-1118

[37] Badhiwala JH, Blackham JR, Bhardwaj RD. Neuropsychiatric changes following penetrating head injury in children. Surgical Neurology International. 2014;**5**:154-154

[38] Kazim SF et al. Management of penetrating brain injury. Journal of Emergencies, Trauma, and Shock. 2011;**4**(3):395-402

[39] Marut D et al. Evaluation of prophylactic antibiotics in penetrating brain injuries at an academic level 1 trauma center. Clinical Neurology and Neurosurgery. 2020;**193**:105777

[40] Heiferman DM, Hayward DM, Ashley WW Jr. Bilateral through-and-through trajectory of a low-velocity transcranial penetrating foreign object in a twelve-month-old. Pediatric Neurosurgery. 2016;**51**(1):25-29

[41] Levy ML et al. Outcome prediction after penetrating Craniocerebral injury in a civilian population: Aggressive surgical Management in Patients with admission Glasgow coma scale scores of 3, 4, or 5. Neurosurgery. 1994;**35**(1):77-85

[42] Levy ML et al. The significance of subarachnoid Hemorrhage after penetrating Craniocerebral injury: Correlations with angiography and outcome in a civilian population. Neurosurgery. 1993;**32**(4):532-540

[43] Diaz A et al. Trauma-induced arterial aneurysm in childhood. Report of a case and review of the literature. Neurochirurgie. 1998;**44**(1):46-49

[44] Levy ML. Economic, ethical, and outcome-based decisions regarding aggressive surgical Management in Patients with Penetrating Craniocerebral Injury. Journal of Health Communication. 1996;**1**(3):301-308

[45] O'Brien NF, Maa T, Yeates KO. The epidemiology of vasospasm in children with moderate-to-severe traumatic brain injury*. Critical Care Medicine. 2015;**43**(3):674-685

[46] Kordestani RK et al. Cerebral arterial spasm after penetrating craniocerebral gunshot wounds: Transcranial Doppler and cerebral blood flow findings. Neurosurgery. 1997;**41**(2):351-359 discussion 359-360

[47] Almojuela A et al. Vasospasm following low-velocity penetrating pediatric intracranial trauma. Journal of Medical Case Reports. 2022;**16**(1):48

Chapter 5

Traumatic Optic Neuropathy

Ainat Klein and Wahbi Wahbi

Abstract

Traumatic optic neuropathy (TON) is a specific neurological sequence of traumatic brain injury (TBI). It has a different mechanism than other most neurologic complications of head trauma and its consequences can be devastating. The damage can be from direct penetrating trauma or bone fracture injuring the optic nerve directly or secondary to indirect blunt trauma (usually causing traction). The diagnosis of TON is based on the clinical history and examination findings indicative of optic neuropathy, especially the presence of defective pupillary light response. TON can cause only mild vision loss but, in some cases, severe vision loss is present. Imaging findings can support the diagnosis, and provide information on the mechanism as well as treatment options. The treatment options include observation alone, systemic steroids, erythropoietin, surgical decompression of the optic canal, or combination. The evidence base for these various treatment options is controversial and each treatment has its side effects and risks. Poor prognostic factors include poor visual acuity at presentation, loss of consciousness, no improvement in vision in the first 48 hours, and evidence of optic canal fractures on neuroimaging.

Keywords: trauma, optic neuropathy, vision loss, steroids, erythropoietin

1. Introduction

Traumatic optic neuropathy (TON) is an acute injury of the optic nerve secondary to blunt or penetrating head injuries, in which dysfunction of the optic nerve, vision impairment, is caused secondary to direct or indirect trauma to the nerve. Traumatic optic neuropathy can be isolated but usually, it is part of more widespread head trauma. Historic studies report an incidence of 0.5–2% of head injuries [1, 2]. A recent national epidemiological survey of TON in the UK found a minimum prevalence in the general population of 1 in 1,000,000 [3].

TON might be present after vehicle accidents (car and bicycle), falls from heights, falling debris, assault, stab, and gunshot wounds (**Figure 1**). Iatrogenic injuries are also reported (mainly secondary to endoscopic sinus surgeries or suprasellar neurosurgeries) [3]. It is important to note that all patients with TON have head injuries and 66% of them have a significant head injury [4]. TON can be present after apparently otherwise mild injuries, but it is most common in the setting of craniofacial fractures [5].

The vast majority of affected patients are young males (79–85%) in their early thirties. Children constitute a large portion as about 20% of patients are younger than 18 years [6]. In this age group, falls (50%) and motor vehicle accidents (40%) are the most common causes of TON.

TON is classified as direct when the nerve is injured directly by a projectile object that penetrates the orbit to damage the optic nerve, or indirect injury when it results from the non-penetrating effects of trauma.

The mechanism of TON is multifactorial. In the case of direct TON damage is caused directly to the nerve by laceration or impingement of the nerve from various causes, including penetrating a foreign body, displaced bone fragment, or optic canal fracture (**Figure 1**). In indirect trauma, compression forces from the superior orbital rim are transferred and concentrated in the orbital roof and optic canal, where the nerve is most vulnerable since it is fixed within the bony optic canal; Coup-contrecoup forces whip mobile portions of the optic nerve against fixed structures, causing injury [7, 8]. Shearing injury to the axons and microvasculature can also play a role, leading to necrosis [9, 10]. Violent rotation of the globe can also result in partial or complete optic nerve avulsion (**Figure 2**) [11]. Depending on the nature of the event, the shock wave can also fracture the optic canal and bone fragments can impinge on the nerve, [8] (occasionally being referred to as direct injury). Diffuse axonal injury is another mechanism that is thought to be involved in TON. As previously reported [12, 13], following head injury, axons of the brain white matter are deformed, swelling, cytoskeleton damage, and impaired axoplasmic transmission led to the disconnection of axons, regression, reorganization, and degeneration.

Orbital compartment syndrome (OCS), in which acute severe bleeding is maintained within the orbit, is another specific subgroup of TON. The orbit is a confined, cone-shaped space, which is bound on all sides by bony walls, except anteriorly, where it is limited by the orbital septum and tarsal plates of the upper and lower eyelid. These structures have limited elasticity and thereby the orbit has limited compliance. Any increase in the orbital content, secondary to bleeding blood vessels, or trapped air, will result in an increase in intra-orbital pressure [14]. Besides

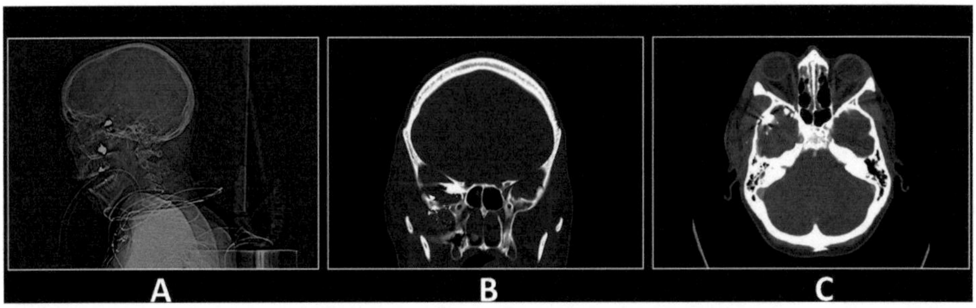

Figure 1.
A 37-year-old female was admitted after gunshot wounds. Upon admission, she was intubated and unconscious. She had multi-compartment hemorrhages, parenchymal, subdural, and subarachnoid and secondary mass effect with midline displacement to the left (not shown). In plain radiograph (A) two metallic foreign bodies were seen. The bottom one is in the right maxillary sinus, with hyperdense small fragments in its track. The second one is adjacent to the right orbital apex. Lateral orbital wall fractures, as well as apical fractures, were noted (B + C). On the first ophthalmologic evaluation, she had pinpoint pupils (secondary to sedative agents) but still, a right RAPD was documented. It was not possible to have dilated fundus exam (DFE). She had no signs of orbital compartment syndrome (no proptosis, free eye movements, and normal intraocular pressure). Multidisciplinary consultation of neurosurgeon, oculoplastic surgeon and ENT, concluded that any surgical intervention aimed to remove the apical foreign body will have a high risk of bleeding and life-threatening complications—It was decided on conservative follow up. Endoscopic sinus surgery was done, removing the maxillary sinus foreign body. Upon regaining consciousness, the patient was evaluated again and had a vision of 20/30 and nonspecific visual field defects. DFE was unremarkable. On her 2 months follow-up, there was no RAPD, and vision improved to 20/20 with no visual field defects.

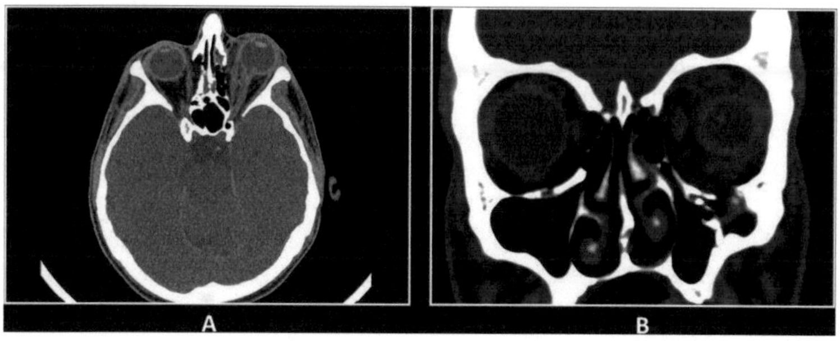

Figure 2.
A 39-year-old male suffered from severe trauma from a surfboard. On first evaluation, he had lacerations of the inferior and superior eyelids with limited eye movements in elevation, suppression and adduction. He had a dilated unresponsive pupil on the left and a vision of NLP in his left eye with RAPD+4. DFE revealed vitreous hemorrhage, and the optic nerve could not be identified in the posterior pole. Besides medial and inferior orbital wall fractures with down displacement into the maxillary sinus (B), the intraconal orbital fat appeared infiltrated and the left optic nerve was thickened and irregular in its course (A). Discontinuity of the posterior aspect of the globe, adjacent to the optic nerve head was noted. A diagnosis of optic nerve avulsion was made, and it was unfortunately impossible to regain vision in this case. Attempts were made to reconstruct the orbit by suturing the lacerations involving the medial cantal folds with excellent cosmetic results, which were important for a young patient.

the possibility of direct compressing on the nerve, it results in disturbing the orbital blood flow and thereby causes acute ischemic damage to the nerve [14, 15].

Post-injury, biochemical cascades exacerbate the initial damage and different treatment modalities are intended to limit this secondary injury. Most cases of visual loss are immediate; however, delayed visual loss is documented in 10% of cases.

2. Diagnosis

Since TON can develop even due to minor head trauma, it should be suspected if any evidence of impaired vision exists following head or facial trauma. In the conscious patient, a detailed history accounting for the mechanism of injury and previous visual status is mandatory. Visual function assessment and comprehensive eye examination should be carried out ruling out other causes of visual loss.

Clinical signs supporting the diagnosis of optic neuropathy include: 1) Impaired visual acuity: about 40–60% of patients present with only light perception vision, or worse [3, 16, 17], although, the visual acuity may range from normal to no light perception. Late deterioration of vision may occur secondary to intra-sheath hematoma and should raise again the diagnosis of TON [16]. 2) Relative afferent pupilar defect (RAPD), an asymmetrical pupillary response to light, which is a very specific sign of optic neuropathy, is very important in the assessment of TON patients; it may be the only subjective evidence at presentation in mild cases and more importantly in the unconscious patient and nonverbal children. A negative RAPD due to symmetric optic nerve injury should always be considered [2]. To note, in the settings of head trauma some patients may have dilated pupils which interferes with the pupillary examination. Alcohol, illicit drugs, narcotics, paralyzing agents, hypothermia, oculomotor nerve neuropathy, and sympathetic injury (Horner's syndrome), can all interfere with pupillary testing [18]. 3) Color vision impairment indicating optic neuropathy.

Visual field defect with variable field defects is another helpful adjunct in the diagnosis and monitoring of TON patients. Unfortunately, in the acute setting, many trauma patients are unable to cooperate and have formal computerized visual field exams.

Visual evoked potentials (VEP) are another important tool in the diagnosis of TON in unconscious and nonverbal patients, providing evidence of visual pathway status and predicting the visual outcome. Patients with better VEP amplitudes have favorable visual outcomes [19].

The optic disc appearance in the early course of TON depends on the site of injury along with the optic nerve. When the injury is anterior to the entry site of the CRA a swollen optic disc with retinal hemorrhages is expected. However, in the majority of the patients, the disc appearance is normal since most of the cases have a more posterior injury. Late in the course of TON, a clinically evident optic atrophy usually develops within 4–6 weeks following the trauma. Kanamori et al. demonstrated that RNFL thinning and RGC complex loss began 2 weeks after trauma and plateaued at 20 weeks [20].

Radiologic studies (CT and MRI) may demonstrate bony fractures, optic sheath hematoma or intra-orbital air, and bleeding (orbital compartment). CT scan with coronal reconstruction images is an excellent imaging modality for demonstrating optic canal fractures [13–15, 21–23]. Multiplayer spiral computed tomographic (MSCT) with spatial stereo reconstruction is an advanced imaging tool that can better evaluate the optic canal status and diagnose combined injuries in other craniofacial tissues [24]. Nevertheless, the role of neuroimaging in the diagnosis of TON is still controversial since the majority of TON patients do not demonstrate relevant findings and the diagnosis can be made on clinical grounds only. However, in a patient with progressive visual loss, repeated neuroimaging is crucial for identifying surgical candidates and directing the surgical treatment.

3. Treatment

Currently, the most common treatments used for TON include 1) systemic steroids; 2) surgical optic nerve decompression; 3) a combination of steroids and surgical decompression. Nevertheless, the treatment of TON remains controversial as spontaneous visual improvement occurs in about 25–50% of TON patients [25, 26]. On the other hand, no medical or surgical treatment was proved until now with a clear advantage over observation only.

Systemic steroid therapy for TON has been extrapolated from the National Acute Spinal Cord Injury Study (NASCIS), a randomized controlled trial comparing steroid treatment to placebo for acute spinal injury, in which increased recovery of neurological function was seen in patients treated with methylprednisolone [27]. The rationale for their use in the treatment of TON is their anti-inflammatory and anti-oxidative effect. Typically, a regimen of very high (megadose) intravenous methylprednisolone is used to treat TON followed by oral steroid with tapering down. The International Optic Nerve Trauma Study (IONTS) is the largest comparative study comparing systemic steroids to surgical decompression and observation using different dosing and timing regimens failed to show any significant difference between the three groups [16]. In addition, there was no clear benefit for any timing or dosage regimen of corticosteroids on the final visual outcome. Lai et al. analyzed the risk factors for visual outcome in a small series of 20 TON patients with initial visual acuity of NLP and found that patients treated with methylprednisolone less than 24 hours from the injury showed better final visual acuity [28]. In another series, Sitaula et al. compared observation to oral prednisone (1 mg/kg for 7 days with 6 weeks taper) and high-dose intravenous methylprednisolone (1 g/d for 3 days followed by oral prednisone taper) found significant visual improvement in the high-dose group compared to the other two groups [29].

Other authors compared different regimes of steroids to observation only did not find any significant difference between their study groups [30–34]. Accounting for their side effects, in the lack of clear effects on visual recovery, steroids should be used judiciously by clinicians. Moreover, a large percentage of TON patients have a concomitant head injury; the CRASH study tested the effectiveness of corticosteroids following acute head injury was terminated prematurely due to an increased mortality rate in patients treated with steroids [35].

3.1 Systemic steroids

Surgical treatment for TON aims to reduce compression on the optic nerve exerted by edema, hematoma, or bony fragments. Currently, the main surgical approaches performed are medial transorbital external ethmoidectomy; transcranial surgery; and endoscopic transnasal surgery [36–38]. The transorbital ethmoidectomy and transcranial approach provide excellent surgical access to the optic canal, however, both are abandoned by many surgeons due to the high rate of complications and undesired cosmetic results. The endoscopic transnasal approach is more commonly used by surgeons. It provides adequate exposure for the medial bony wall of the optic canal through the sphenoid sinus with a less invasive procedure and more acceptable cosmetic results. However, it is a high-risk procedure due to the proximity of the internal carotid artery to the optic canal; and it should be done only by highly experienced surgeons in this kind of surgery. Several studies reporting the results of surgical decompression with or without steroids had been published in the literature with visual improvement rates ranging from 18–81% [39–46]. Since primary reports failed to show obvious benefits for surgical decompression over observation, efforts are still made by researchers to optimize the visual outcomes following surgery. Reasonably, the authors presented the following indications for surgical treatment [23, 42–47]: 1) history of traumatic head or face injury; 2) presence of hematoma or bony fragments compressing the optic verve; 3) poor response to initial medical therapy; 4) progressive visual loss not explained by other nontraumatic ocular pathology; 5) lack of evident damage to ocular tissue or intracranial optic nerve; 6) prolonger latency or reduction of amplitude in preoperative VEP scan. The optimal timing for surgery has been evaluated by several authors based on their own experiences. While some authors reported better visual outcomes in the early surgical intervention (<3 days) [48–50], others reported comparable visual improvement in the late surgical intervention (>7 days) [51]. Yu et al. compared immediate (within 3 days) to delayed (>3 days) optic canal decompression, and found that 73.5% of patients in the immediate surgical decompression group showed improved vision versus 46.9% in the delayed group [36]. Even though, the benefit of surgical decompression or the combination of surgical and medical treatment remains uncertain due to the lack of large comparative controlled studies. Moreover, several surgical complications, including CSF leak, infection, and bleeding, have been reported [37, 52–54]. Therefore, in the lack of clear evidence, the potential benefits and drawbacks of surgical treatment should be discussed in detail with the patient before surgery.

3.2 Surgical treatment

In cases suspected of OCS, the examination must be performed as soon as possible, so as not to delay treatment. The conscious patient will complain about severe pain and vision loss. The patient will usually have marked eyelid swelling, proptosis, chemosis, and even subconjunctival hemorrhage. Severe ophthalmoplegia will be noted and even digital ocular palpation will demonstrate resistance to retropulsion and a firm globe indicating an elevated IOP. CT may be helpful in establishing the diagnosis in milder cases where there is uncertainty and vision remains intact, but when the clinical findings are suggestive and vision is markedly impaired, treatment should not be postponed until after imaging is performed. In cases of OCS urgent surgical decompression is the mainstay of treatment. A bedside, lateral canthotomy and cantholysis (LC/C) is the first-line approach for reducing intra-orbital pressure [55]. Bony orbital decompression can be considered an adjuvant procedure if an adequate response is not achieved after LC/C [56]. In these cases, reviewing orbital imaging is important to locate the hematoma or other causative pathology (air, abscess), and to plane the surgical approach (endonasal medial wall decompression, anterior orbitotomy via an eyelid crease incision, or transcranial approach) [14].

3.3 Erythropoietin

In the last few years, erythropoietin was suggested as a potential treatment for TON due to its anti-inflammatory and antiapoptotic effects, based on studies of CNS trauma patients [57]. Primary studies reported better visual outcomes with EPO treatment [58, 59]. Recently, the TONTT, a phase 3, a large comparative study compared erythropoietin to steroids and observation in 100 TON patients [60]. All three study groups demonstrated significant visual improvement compared to the baseline BCVA. However, no significant difference was found between the study groups. Of note, color vision improvement was also observed in all three study groups even though it was significant only in the erythropoietin group.

3.4 Experimental treatments

In the last two decades, research is ongoing to develop new therapies aiming to encourage neuroprotection and axonal regeneration. Stem cell transplantation is gaining more progress in the treatment of optic nerve damage due to their multidirectional differentiation. In a mice model, stem cells transplanted in the subretinal space differentiated into photoreceptor and retinal cells [61].

Recently, a prospective single-center prospective phase 1 study, investigated mesenchymal stem cell (MSC) transplantation in 20 patients with traumatic optic neuropathy. Optic canal decompression with mesenchymal stem cell implantation compared to optic canal decompression alone. Both groups showed significant improvements in vision compared with the baseline; however, there was no statistically significant difference between the study groups [62].

Investigations on other potential therapies, including anti-TNF, brain-derived neurotrophic factor (BDNF), and RNA, aiming to reduce retinal ganglion cell loss and encouraging axonal regeneration are in progress [63–65].

Currently, no standard of care therapy exists in addressing TON.

4. Prognosis

Spontaneous visual recovery of about 40–60% has been reported in TON patients treated conservatively [9]. The final visual acuity following TON has a wide range from 20/20 to NLP [28, 29]. The baseline visual acuity is the most important prognostic factor for recovery since it reflects the degree of damage to the optic nerve. Patients with better visual function are presumed to have more functioning retinal ganglion cells, while patients with no residual vision and poor visual acuity at a presentation associated have less functioning retinal ganglion cells. Hence, better visual acuity at presentation predicts a better final visual outcome, on the contrary, patients with no residual vision (NLP) have lower final visual outcomes.

According to some reports, patients who present with NLP are unlikely to improve at all [29, 66–68], while other reports indicated some rate of improvement even in a patient with no residual vision at presentation [66]. In patients with residual vision, those with lower visual acuity at presentation sometimes show more visual improvement rates [68–70]. Other negative prognostic factors presented by different authors include lack of improvement within the first 48 hours, optic canal fracture, absence of VEP responses, loss of consciousness, higher degrees of RAPD, age over 40 years, intra-sheath hematoma, and blood within the posterior ethmoidal cells [19, 71–73].

In cases of OCS, if treated within 2 hours, most patients will achieve a final visual acuity better than 20/40, though approximately 15% will be worse. Patients treated after 2 hours have poorer reported outcomes. In the case of delayed presentation, considering orbital decompression is still reasonable since there are reports of visual recovery even after delayed intervention and even with no decompression at all [74].

It is important to emphasize that recovery of vision after any kind of treatment modality mentioned, is not always immediate. There may be an ongoing improvement in VA for a few weeks post-intervention. Furthermore, most reports published provide a limited follow-up period and it is reasonable to deduce that long-term follow-up may show better outcomes. It should also be noted that even in cases of good VA acuity, some patients suffer from severe visual field defects.

Author details

Ainat Klein* and Wahbi Wahbi
Department of Ophthalmology, Tel Aviv Suaraski Medical Center, Tel Aviv University, Tel Aviv, Israel

*Address all correspondence to: kleinainat@gmail.com

References

[1] Steinsapir KD, Goldberg RA. Traumatic optic neuropathy. Survey of Ophthalmology. 1994;**38**:487-518

[2] Cockerham GC, Goodrich GL, Weichel LED, et al. Eye and visual function in traumatic brain injury. The Journal of Rehabilitation Research and Development. 2009;**46**(6):811-818

[3] Lee V, Ford RL, Xing W, Bunce C, Foot B. Surveillance of traumatic optic neuropathy in the UK. Eye (London, England). 2010;**24**(2):240-250

[4] Pirouzmand F. Epidemiological trends of traumatic optic nerve injuries in the largest Canadian adult trauma center. Journal of Craniofacial Surgery. 2012;**23**(2):516-520

[5] Jamal BT, Pfahler SM, Lane KA, et al. Ophthalmic injuries in patients with zygomaticomaxillary complex fractures requiring surgical repair. Journal of Oral and Maxillofacial Surgery. 2009;**67**:986-989

[6] Goldenberg-Cohen N, Miller NR, Repka MX. Traumatic optic neuropathy in children and adolescents. Journal of American Association for Pediatric Ophthalmology and Strabismus. 2004;**8**:20-27

[7] Gross CE, Dekock JR, Panje WR, Hershkowitz N, Newman J. Evidence for orbital deformation that may contribute to monocular blindness following minor frontal head trauma. Journal of Neurosurgery. 1981;**55**:963-966

[8] Crompton MR. Visual lesions in closed head injury. Brain. 1970;**93**:785-792

[9] Walsh FB, Hoyt WF. Clinical Neuro-Ophthalmology. 3rd ed. Vol. 3. Baltimore: Williams & Wilkins; 1969. p. 2380

[10] Thale A, Jungmann K, Paulsen F. Morphological studies of the optic canal. Orbit. 2002;**21**(2):131-137

[11] Foster BS, March GA, Lucarelli MJ, Samiy N, Lessell S. Optic nerve avulsion. Archives of Ophthalmology. 1997;**115**(5):623-630

[12] Smith DH, Meaney DF. Axonal damage in traumatic brain injury. The Neuroscientist. 2000;**6**(6):483-495

[13] Wang J, Hamm RJ, Povlishock JT. Traumatic axonal injury in the optic nerve: Evidence for axonal swelling, disconnection, dieback, and reorganization. Journal of Neurotrauma. 2011;**28**(7):1185-1198

[14] McCallum E, Keren S, Lapira M, Norris JH. Orbital compartment syndrome: An update with review of the literature. Clinical Ophthalmology. 2019;**13**:2189-2194

[15] Hargaden M, Goldberg SH, Cunningham D, Breton ME, Griffith JW, Lang CM. Optic neuropathy following simulation of orbital hemorrhage in the nonhuman primate. Ophthalmic Plastic and Reconstructive Surgery. 1996;**12**(4):264-272

[16] Levin LA, Beck RW, Joseph MP, Seiff S, Kraker R. The treatment of traumatic optic neuropathy — The international optic nerve trauma study. Ophthalmology. 1999;**106**:1268

[17] Lessell S. Indirect optic-nerve trauma. Archives of Ophthalmology. 1989;**107**:382-386

[18] Meyer S, Gibb T, Jurkovich GJ. Evaluation and significance of the pupillary light reflex in trauma patients.

Annals of Emergency Medicine. 1993;**22**(6):1052-1057

[19] Tabatabaei SA, Soleimani M, Alizadeh M, et al. Predictive value of visual evoked potentials, relative afferent pupillary defect, and orbital fractures in patients with traumatic optic neuropathy. Clinical Ophthalmology. 2011;**5**:1021-1026

[20] Kanamori A, Nakamura M, Yamada Y, Negi A. Longitudinal study of retinal nerve Fiber layer thickness and ganglion cell complex in traumatic optic neuropathy. Archives of Ophthalmology. 2012;**130**(8):1067-1069

[21] Guyon JJ, Brant-Zawadzki M, Seiff SR. CT demonstration of optic canal fractures. AJR. 1984;**143**:1031-1103

[22] Ibanez L, Navallas M, de Caceres IA, Martinez-Chamorro E, Borruel S. CT features of posttraumatic vision loss. AJR. American Journal of Roentgenology. 2021;**217**(2):469-479

[23] Manfredi SJ, Raji MR, Sprinkle PM, Weinstein GW, Minardi LM, Swanson TJ. Computerized tomographic scan findings in facial fractures associated with blindness. Plastic and Reconstructive Surgery. 1981;**68**(4):479-490

[24] Yang Q, Li Y, Zou Y, et al. Computer-assisted three-dimensional reconstruction and spatial stereotaxis study of optic canal with multiplayer spiral computed tomographic. Neurosurgical Review. 2008;**22**:306-308 311

[25] Wang BH, Robertson BC, Girotto JA, et al. Traumatic optic neuropathy: A review of 61 patients. Plastic and Reconstructive Surgery. 2001;**107**(7):1655-1664

[26] Jang SY. Traumatic optic neuropathy. Korean Journal of Neurotrauma. 2018;**14**(1):1-5

[27] Bracken MB, Shepard MJ, Collins WF, et al. A randomized, controlled trial of methylprednisolone or naloxone in the treatment of acute spinal-cord injury. Results of the second national acute spinal cord injury study. The New England Journal of Medicine. 1990;**322**(20):1405-1411

[28] Lai IL, Liao HT, Chen CT. Risk factors analysis for the outcome of indirect traumatic optic neuropathy with steroid pulse therapy. Annals of Plastic Surgery. 2016;**76**(Suppl 1):6

[29] Sitaula S, Dahal HN, Sharma AK. Clinical evaluation and treatment outcome of traumatic optic neuropathy in Nepal: A retrospective case series. Neuro-Ophthalmology. 2017;**42**(1):17-24

[30] Carta A, Ferrigno L, Leaci R, et al. Long-term outcome after conservative treatment of indirect traumatic optic neuropathy. European Journal of Ophthalmology. 2006;**16**:847-850

[31] Lee KF, Muhd Nor NI, Yaakub A, Wan Hitam W. Traumatic optic neuropathy: A review of 24 patients. International Journal of Ophthalmology. 2010;**3**:175-178

[32] Entezari M, Rajavi Z, Sedighi N, et al. High-dose intravenous methylprednisolone in recent traumatic optic neuropathy: A randomized double-masked placebo-controlled clinical trial. Graefe's Archive for Clinical and Experimental Ophthalmology. 2007;**245**:1267-1271

[33] Yu-Wai-Man P, Griffiths PG. Steroids for traumatic optic neuropathy. Cochrane Database of Systematic Reviews. 2013;**6**:CD006032

[34] Chaon BC, Lee MS. Is there treatment for traumatic optic neuropathy? Current Opinion in Ophthalmology. 2015;**26**(6):445-449

[35] CRASH Trial Collaborators. Final results of MRC CRASH, a rFandomised placebo-controlled trial of intravenous corticosteroid in adults with head injury-outcomes at 6 months. Lancet. 2005;**365**(9475):1957-1959

[36] Yu B, Ma Y, Tu Y, Wu W. The outcome of endoscopic transethmosphenoid optic canal decompression for indirect traumatic optic neuropathy with no-light-perception. Journal of Ophthalmology. 2016;**2016**:6492858

[37] Yan W, Chen Y, Qian Z, et al. Incidence of optic canal fracture in the traumatic optic neuropathy and its effect on the visual outcome. The British Journal of Ophthalmology. 2017;**101**:261-267

[38] Chen HH, Lee MC, Tsai CH, et al. Surgical decompression or corticosteroid treatment of indirect traumatic optic neuropathy: A randomized controlled trial. Annals of Plastic Surgery. 2020;**84**:S80-S83

[39] Chen M, Jiang Y, Pang WH, et al. A 212 cases analysis of treatment for traumatic optic europathy by nasal endoscopic optic nerve decompression. Lin Chung Er Bi Yan Hou Tou Jing Wai Ke Za Zhi. 2017;**31**:1411-1414

[40] Gupta AK, Gupta AK, Gupta A, et al. Traumatic optic neuropathy in pediatric population: Early intervention or delayed intervention? International Journal of Pediatric Otorhinolaryngology. 2007;**71**:559-562

[41] Peng A, Li Y, Hu P, et al. Endoscopic optic nerve decompression for traumatic optic neuropathy in children. International Journal of Pediatric Otorhinolaryngology. 2011;**75**:992-998

[42] Sun J, Cai X, Zou W, et al. Outcome of endoscopic optic nerve decompression for traumatic optic neuropathy. The Annals of Otology, Rhinology, and Laryngology. 2021;**130**:56-59

[43] Wladis EJ, Aakalu VK, Sobel RK, et al. Interventions for indirect traumatic optic neuropathy: A report by the American Academy of ophthalmology. Ophthalmology. 2021;**128**(6):928-937

[44] Yang QT, Zhang GH, Liu X, Ye J, Li Y. The therapeutic efficacy of endoscopic optic nerve decompression and its effects on the prognoses of 96 cases of traumatic optic neuropathy. Journal of Trauma and Acute Care Surgery. 2012;**72**:1350-1355

[45] Oh H-J, Yeo D-G, Hwang S-C. Surgical treatment for traumatic optic neuropathy. Korean Journal of Neurotrauma. 2018;**14**(2):55-60

[46] Gupta D, Gadodia M. Transnasal endoscopic optic nerve decompression in post traumatic optic neuropathy. Indian Journal of Otolaryngology and Head & Neck Surgery. 2018;**70**:49-52

[47] Otani N, Wada K, Fujii K, Toyooka T, Kumagai K, Ueno H, et al. Usefulness of extradural optic nerve decompression via trans-superior orbital fissure approach for treatment of traumatic optic nerve injury: Surgical procedures and techniques from experience with 8 consecutive patients. World Neurosurgery. 2016;**90**:357-363

[48] Emanuelli E, Bignami M, Digilio E, Fusetti S, Volo T, Castelnuovo P. Post-traumatic optic neuropathy: Our surgical and medical protocol. European Archives of Oto-Rhino-Laryngology. 2015;**272**(11):3301-3309

[49] Wohlrab TM, Maas S, de Carpentier JP. Surgical decompression in traumatic optic neuropathy. Acta Ophthalmologica Scandinavica. 2002;**80**:287-293

[50] Martinez-Perez R, Albonette-Felicio T, Hardesty DA, et al. Outcome of the surgical decompression for traumatic optic neuropathy: A systematic review and meta-analysis. Neurosurgical Review. Apr 2021;**44**(2):633-641

[51] Dhaliwal SS, Sowerby LJ, Rotenberg BW. Timing of endoscopic surgical decompression in traumatic optic neuropathy: A systematic review of the literature. International Forum of Allergy & Rhinology. 2016;**6**:661-667

[52] He Z, Li Q, Yuan J, et al. Evaluation of transcranial surgical decompression of the optic canal as a treatment option for traumatic optic neuropathy. Clinical Neurology and Neurosurgery. 2015;**134**:130-135

[53] Li H, Zhou B, Shi J, et al. Treatment of traumatic optic neuropathy: Our experience of endoscopic optic nerve decompression. The Journal of Laryngology and Otology. 2008;**122**:1325-1329

[54] Li HB, Shi JB, Cheng L, et al. Salvage optic nerve decompression for traumatic blindness under nasal endoscopy: Risk and benefit analysis. Clinical Otolaryngology. 2007;**32**:447-451

[55] Haubner F, Jägle H, Nunes DP, et al. Orbital compartment: Effects of emergent canthotomy and cantholysis. European Archives of Oto-Rhino-Laryngology. 2015;**272**(2):479-483

[56] Lee KYC, Tow S, Fong K-S. Visual recovery following emergent orbital decompression in traumatic retrobulbar haemorrhage. Annals of the Academy of Medicine, Singapore. 2006;**35**(11):831-832

[57] Ghezzi P, Brines M. Erythropoietin as an antiapoptotic, tissue-protective cytokine. Cell Death and Differentiation. 2004;**11**(Suppl 1):S37-S44

[58] Kashkouli MB, Pakdel F, Sanjari MS et al.) Erythropoietin: A novel treatment for traumatic optic neuropathy—A pilot study: Graefe's Archive for Clinical and Experimental Ophthalmology 2011;**249**(5):731-736

[59] Entezari M, Esmaeili M, Yaseri M. A pilot study of the effect of intravenous erythropoetin on improvement of visual function in patients with recent indirect traumatic optic neuropathy. Graefe's Archive for Clinical and Experimental Ophthalmology. 2014;**252**(8): 1309-1313

[60] Kashkouli MB, Yousefi S, Nojomi M, et al. Traumatic optic neuropathy treatment trial (TONTT): Open label, phase 3, multicenter, semi-experimental trial. Graefe's Archive for Clinical and Experimental Ophthalmology. 2018;**256**:209-218

[61] Feng X, Chen P, Zhao X, et al. Transplanted embryonic retinal stem cells have the potential to repair the injured retina in mice. BMC Ophthalmology. 2021;**21**:26

[62] Li J, Bai X, Guan X, Yuan H, Xu X. Treatment of Optic Canal decompression combined with umbilical cord mesenchymal stem (stromal) cells for indirect traumatic optic neuropathy: A phase 1 clinical trial. Ophthalmic Research. 2021;**64**(3):398-404

[63] Tse BC, Dvoriantchikova G, Tao W, et al. Tumor necrosis factor inhibition in the acute management of traumatic optic neuropathy. Investigative Ophthalmology & Visual Science. 2018;**59**:2905-2912

[64] Cui Q, So KF, Yip HK. Major biological effects of neurotrophic factors on retinal ganglion cells in mammals. Biological Signals and Receptors. 1998;**7**:220-226

[65] Park KK, Liu K, Hu Y, et al. Promoting axon regeneration in the adult CNS by modulation of the PTEN/mTOR pathway. Science. 2008;**322**:963-966

[66] Yu B, Chen Y, Ma Y, Tu Y, Wu W. Outcome of endoscopic trans-ethmosphenoid optic canal decompression for indirect traumatic optic neuropathy in children. BMC Ophthalmology. 2008;**18**(1):152

[67] Steinsapir KD. Treatment of traumatic optic neuropathy with high-dose corticosteroid. Journal of Neuro-Ophthalmology. 2006;**26**:65-67

[68] Yang WG, Chen CT, Tsay PK, de Villa GH, Tsai YJ, Chen YR. Outcome for traumatic optic neuropathy--surgical versus nonsurgical treatment. Annals of Plastic Surgery. 2004;**52**(1):36-42

[69] Ma YJ, Yu B, Tu YH, et al. Prognostic factors of transethmosphenoid optic canal decompression for indirect traumatic optic neuropathy. International Journal of Ophthalmology. 2018;**11**:1222-1226

[70] Song Y, Li H, Ma Y, et al. Analysis of prognostic factors of endoscopic optic nerve decompression in traumatic blindness. Acta Oto-Laryngologica. 2013;**133**:1196-1200

[71] Holmes Mark D, Sires Bryan S. Flash visual evoked potentials predict visual outcome in traumatic optic neuropathy. Ophthalmic Plastic & Reconstructive Surgery. 2004;**20**(5):342-346

[72] Mohammed MA, Mossallam E, Allam IY. The role of the flash visual evoked potential in evaluating visual function in patients with indirect traumatic optic neuropathy. Clinical Ophthalmology. 2021;**30**(15): 1349-1355

[73] Carta A, Ferrigno L, Salvo M, Bianchi-Marzoli S, Boschi A, Carta F. Visual prognosis after indirect traumatic optic neuropathy. Journal of Neurology, Neurosurgery, and Psychiatry. 2003;**74**:246-248

[74] Ujam A, Perry M. Emergency management for orbital compartment syndrome-is decompression mandatory? International Journal of Oral and Maxillofacial Surgery. 2016;**45**(11):1435-1437

Chapter 6

Traumatic Injury of the Carotid and Vertebral Arteries and their Neurointerventional Treatment

Huachen Zhang, Hanrui Xu, Shikai Liang and Xianli Lv

Abstract

Traumatic injuries of the carotid and vertebral arteries include direct carotid-cavernous fistula, intracranial pseudoaneurysm and arterial dissection, which cause a series of symptoms and may be life threatening. Computed tomographic angiography is the most common modality for initial screening and diagnosis. The subsequent management of any identified vessel injury, however, is not clearly defined. With the development of neurointerventional materials and technology, endovascular therapy is playing an important role in treatment of these neurovascular injuries. Balloon, coil, liquid embolic materials, covered stent and flow diversion have been effectively used in clinical practice. This chapter reviews the epidemiology, injury mechanism, clinical manifestations, classification system, diagnostic imaging and endovascular treatment of traumatic neurovascular injuries.

Keywords: carotid artery, vertebral artery, neurointerventional treatment, trauma, vascular injury

1. Introduction

Distribution of traumatic neurovascular injuries by location was 42% intracranial, 39% cervical, and 19% extracranial [1]. For the early recognition of lesions in different locations, imaging and clinical manifestations are the key to diagnosis. With regard to the treatment of these traumatic neurovascular diseases, the paradigm of treatment has shift from the destructive modality of carotid artery ligation or trapping to reconstructive modality of neurointerventional treatment. Endovascular treatment has been the first line treatment for traumatic injuries of the carotid and vertebral arteries including direct carotid-cavernous fistula, intracranial pseudoaneurysm and arterial dissection [1].

2. Traumatic carotid-cavernous fistula

Traumatic carotid-cavernous fistula (TCCF) represents abnormal vascular communications in the skull base between the carotid artery system and the adjacent cavernous sinus [2]. TCCF is the most common type of CCF [3, 4]. Within the

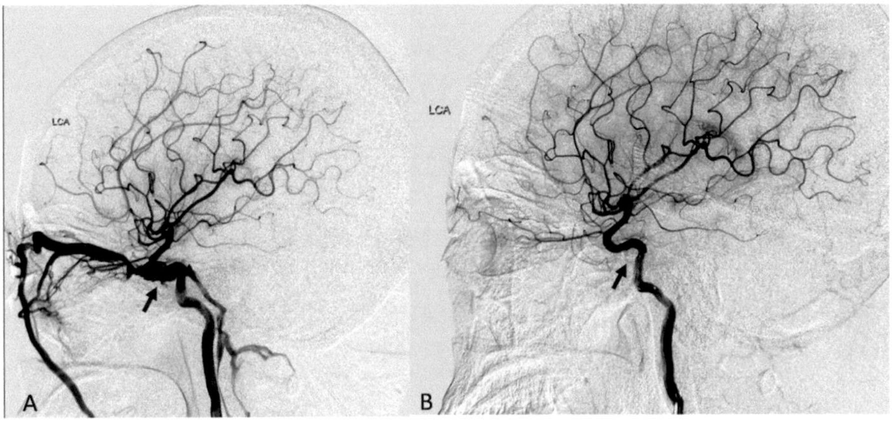

Figure 1.
A woman presented a traumatic CCF treated with detachable coils. A: Lateral view of the left internal carotid artery angiogram showing a direct CCF of Zipfel's type II with ophthalmic vein reflux (arrow). B: Lateral view of the left internal carotid artery angiogram showing complete obliteration of the CCF after coil embolization (arrow).

cavernous sinus, the internal carotid artery (ICA) is bound by strong dural filaments and attachments, especially at its entrance and exit by its inferior and superior ascending segments [5]. Trauma can cause an intima-to-adventitia tearing in the ICA, leading to high-flow shunt between the cavernous sinus portion of the ICA and the cavernous sinus (**Figure 1**) [6]. TCCF also can be caused by iatrogenic injury from neurointerventional therapy, percutaneous treatment of trigeminal neuralgia, or transsphenoidal resection of pituitary tumor [6]. Endovascular recanalization of symptomatic chronic internal carotid artery occlusion (ICAOS) may cause CCF, because during the operation there may be severe ICA dissection with intimal inlet at the proximal end of ICA and adventitial outlet in ICA [6, 7]. In 1985, Barrow and his colleagues developed the classification system after extensive angiographic studies (**Table 1**) [8]. TCCF is of type A in Barrow's classification system. A recent grading system of dural arteriovenous fistulas (DAVFs) was proposed by Zipfel GJ from Washington University in 2009 covering CCFs (**Table 2**) [9]. The Zipfel's classification can stratify clinical status of cerebral and spinal DAVFs according to understanding of natural history in order to guide the appropriate evaluation and therapies of lesions [10].

The clinical manifestations of TCCF are mainly related to venous hypertension or venous rupture. The venous drainage from the cavernous sinus to the superior and inferior ophthalmic veins causes prominent ocular symptoms, such as progressive pulsatile exophthalmos, conjunctival congestion or edema, in 90% patients [5]. In up to 50% patients, visual loss may result from decreased ocular or retinal perfusion and

Type	Feeding arteries
A	the cavernous segment of the internal carotid artery
B	the branch of the internal carotid artery that supplies the dura mater
C	the branch of the external carotid artery that supplies the dura mater
D	the branch of the internal and external carotid artery that supplies the dura mater.

Table 1.
The classification system of CCF introduced by Barrow and his colleagues [8].

Type	Description
I	DAVFs are those that drain into the dural sinus with antegrade venous flow, e.g., the flow of the veins draining from the parenchyma or spinal cord into the dural sinuses or epidural veins is anterograde, a cavernous sinus fistula (CSF) without cortical or ophthalmic vein (OV) drainage.
II	DAVFs drain into dural sinus with retrograde venous flow, a CSF with OV drainage without cortical drainage. Type II DAVFs can drain into spinal perimedullary veins via dural sinuses.
III	DAVFs are those that drain into the pial veins and the spinal coronal or perimedullary veins, including CSF with cortical drainage. Type III can drain into spinal perimedullary veins and Type III spinal DAVFs can drain intracranially via pial veins.

Table 2.
The classification system of dural arteriovenous fistulas (DAVFs) introduced by Zipfel et al. in 2009 [9].

papilledema because of venous stasis [11]. Cranial nerve dysfunction in III, IV, VI can cause diplopia [11]. Intracranial pulsatile tinnitus was obvious in patients with inferior petrosal sinus. The increased venous pressure caused by cortical venous drainage leads to venous rupture and bleeding.

3. Traumatic neurovascular Pseudoaneurysm

Neurovascular pseudoaneurysm formation is the result of partial to complete disruption of the cerebral arterial wall, which ultimately leads to hematoma that is contained by the adventitia of the vessel wall or the perivascular soft tissues [12].

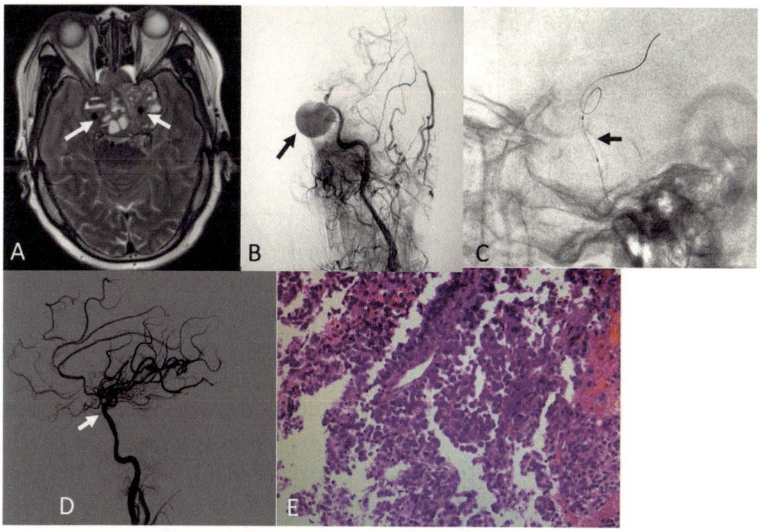

Figure 2.
A 59-year-old woman presented decreased vision in both eyes. A: Axial MR imaging, T2-weighted, showing an invasive pituitary tumor involving bilateral internal carotid arteries (arrows). During transnasal endoscopic pituitary tumor resection, the left internal carotid artery was injured. After hemostasis by tamponade, cerebral angiography was performed for endovascular intervention. B: Frontal view of the left carotid artery angiogram showing a giant pseudoaneurysm of the cavernous segment of the internal carotid artery (arrow). C: Lateral view of the unsubtracted image showing the Willis covered stent was released (arrow). D: Lateral view of the left internal carotid artery angiogram showing complete obliteration of the giant pseudoaneurysm (arrow). E: the histological examination confirmed pituitary adenoma (H-E staining).

Traumatic ICA pseudoaneurysms are rare, mostly occurring in the petrous bone segment and cavernous sinus segment, accounting for less than 1% of all aneurysms [13]. Traffic accidents, stab wounds and falling injuries cause 51%, 12% and 8% of traumatic aneurysms, respectively [14]. The risk factors related to pseudoaneurysm formation mainly include male patient, young age, skull base fracture, intracranial hemorrhage and high-energy injury mechanism [15, 16]. The pressure of arterial pulsation can form pulsatile hematoma, so pseudoaneurysm is easy to rupture. It is reported that most pseudoaneurysms will bleed again 3–7 days after injury, and the mortality rate is as high as 50% [17].

Pseudoaneurysms of carotid and vertebral arteries caused by iatrogenic arterial injury have also been reported. The injury of ICA during the operation of pituitary tumor and complex cervical hypervascular tumor can cause carotid pseudoaneurysm (**Figure 2**). Michael J. Alexander and his colleagues reported a case of acute petrous carotid pseudoaneurysm after myringotomy procedure [18]. Surgical treatment of craniocervical junction lesions may lead to the vertebral artery pseudoaneurysm.

Rupture of intracranial pseudoaneurysm will lead to subarachnoid hemorrhage, and the patient is characterized by severe headache, nausea, vomiting and meningeal irritation [19]. Giant hematoma can compress and damage adjacent nerves and blood vessels, resulting in ischemic symptoms of distal cerebral tissues. Moreover, pseudoaneurysm changes the blood flow, and easily forms thrombus in the aneurysm sac. When the thrombus falls off, it will cause the embolism of the distal artery leading to symptoms of stroke.

4. Traumatic arterial dissection

Dissections of the carotid and vertebral arteries are due to laceration that occur in the intimal layer, which leads to blood under arterial pressure to enter the wall of the vessel and form an intramural hematoma [20]. The incidence of traumatic dissection of the carotid and vertebral arteries has been reported to be 0.08–0.4% of overall traumatic populations [21]. The most common sites of traumatic carotid and vertebral arterial dissections are 2–3 cm from the distal end of the bifurcations of the carotid artery and at C1–2 level, respectively [22]. Iatrogenic neurovascular dissection is a common complication, which is mainly attributed to damage of intimal layer caused by manipulation of guide wire and catheters [23].

Headaches are often the first symptom in adults [24]. Children usually present with symptoms of cerebral ischemia and most commonly hemiparesis [21, 25]. Because children's blood vessel is particularly vulnerable to stretching, and distorting forces. Trauma leads to a traumatic endothelial intimal lesion, followed by fibrin accumulation, leucocyte reaction, and the formation of thrombus to occlude the vascular lumen [26]. In patients presenting with sudden onset of unilateral Horner syndrome, the diagnosis of vertebral arterial dissection should be considered [27].

Early diagnosis of traumatic neurovascular dissection is necessary. Transcranial Doppler, computed tomography (CT), computed tomography angiography (CTA), and magnetic resonance imaging (MRI) can diagnose traumatic neurovascular diseases. Neurovascular dissection can be seen on T1 and T2 weighted images [28, 29]. According to a new study on the diagnosis of dissection, simultaneous non-contrast angiography and intraplaque hemorrhage (SNAP) sequence and T1-weighted volumetric isotropic turbo spin echo acquisition (T1-w VISTA) sequences in MRI can recognize intramural hematoma, intimal flap, and double lumen but SNAP images had significantly higher intramural hematoma wall contrast than T1-w VISTA images. Therefore, SNAP sequence can early diagnose the neurovascular arterial dissection [29]. Cerebral angiography is not only a diagnostic tool, but also the basis of endovascular therapy of cerebrospinal vascular disorders.

5. Neurointerventional treatment

5.1 Traumatic carotid cavernous fistula

With the development of endovascular neurosurgery, neurovascular therapy has become the main treatment of TCCFs [30–33]. In the 1960s and early 1970s, it is known that Serbinenko had developed a detachable, flow-directed balloon that was used to treat TCCF while preserving the carotid artery [33]. In China, detachable balloon was used to treat TCCF since the late of 1980s (**Figures 3** and **4**). Coil embolization may be considered in case of the small fistula (**Figure 1**). Temporary balloon or neurostent can be placed in the parent artery to prevent the coil from falling off and occluding the distal intracranial circulation [31]. But, balloon or coil embolization might cause cranial nerve palsy [32]. The detachable balloon or the application of the coil can occlude the fistula, which can maintain the patency of the ICA of the affected side in 70–90% cases (**Figure 5**) [33]. Transarterial embolization of TCCFs using detachable balloons or coils was considered to be a feasible, effective, and safe method for the treatment [34].

Two liquid embolic agents, n-butyl cyanoacrylate (nBCA) (Codman Neurovascular, Raynham, Massachusetts) and ethylene-vinyl alcohol copolymer (EVOH) (Onyx, ev3, Irvine, California) have become good choices. TCCF can be cured by transvenous catheterization of the cavernous sinus and embolization using Onyx assisted with transient balloon occlusion of the ICA at the fistula site. The Willis covered stent (Micro-Port, Shanghai, China) can protect the parent artery and

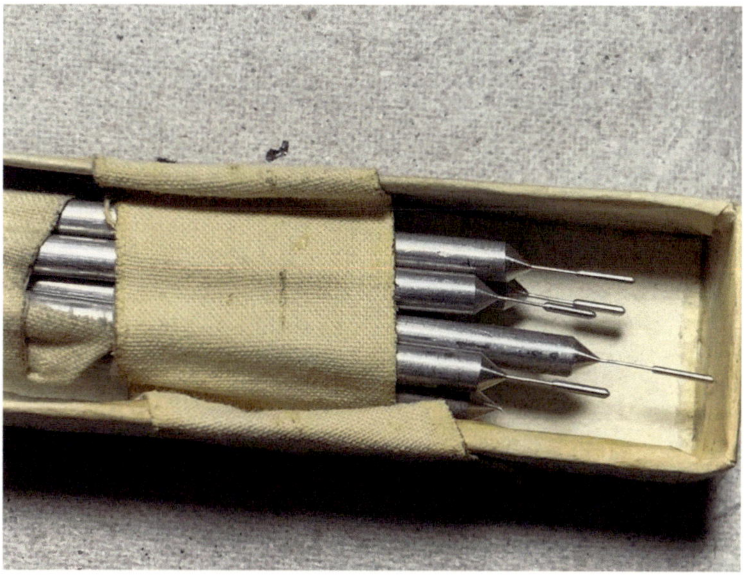

Figure 3.
Molds used by Prof. Zhongxue Wu for making detachabel latex balloons in the year of 1988.

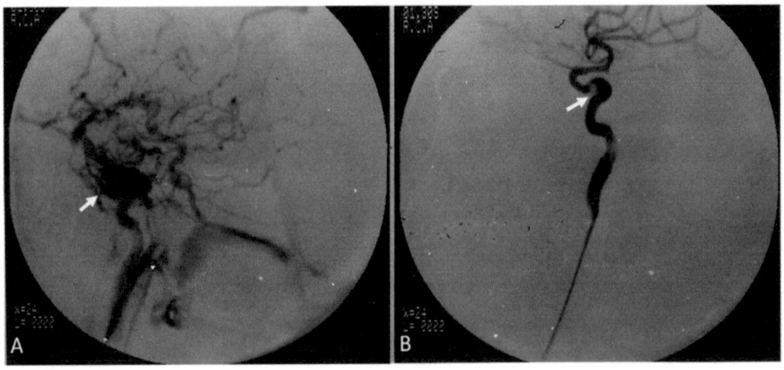

Figure 4.
A 40-year-old man presented a traumatic CCF treated with detachable balloon in the year of 1988. A: Lateral view of internal carotid artery angiogram showing a direct CCF of Zipfel's type III with cortical veins reflux (arrow). B: Lateral view of internal carotid artery angiogram showing complete obliteration of the CCF after balloon embolization (arrow).

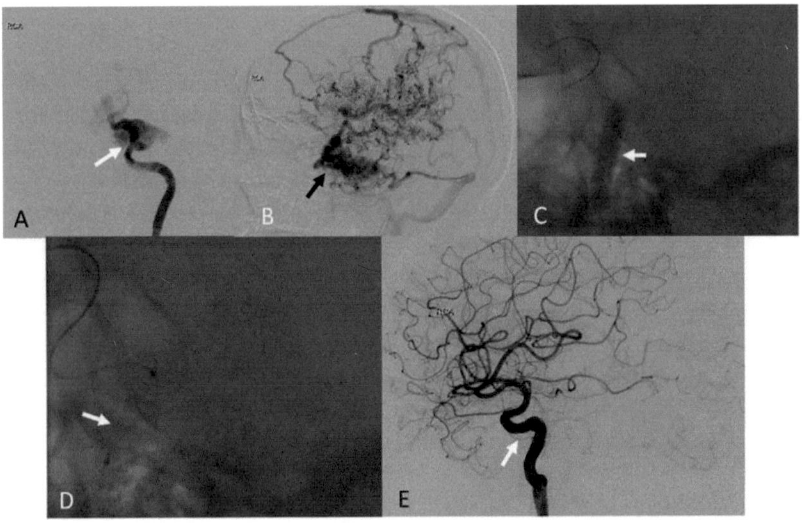

Figure 5.
A 27-year-old man presented a traumatic CCF treated with Willis covered stent. A: Lateral view of the right internal carotid artery angiogram, early arterial phase. B: Lateral view of the right internal carotid artery angiogram, late arterial phase. Showing a direct CCF of Zipfel's type III with pial veins reflux (arrow). C: Lateral view of the unsubtracted image showing the inflation of the balloon(arrow). D, lateral view of the unsubtracted image showing the Willis covered stent was released (arrow). E: Lateral view of the right internal carotid artery angiogram showing complete obliteration of the CCF after treatment (arrow).

the mid- and long-term occlusion rate is reported to be 95.7% (**Figure 6**) [35]. Flow diversion is also an effective treatment. Its principle is that a flow diversion in the parent artery can reduce and disturb blood flow in the aneurismal sac causing blood stagnation and thrombosis [36].

5.2 Neurovascular Pseudoaneurysm

Endovascular treatment for neurovascular pseudoaneurysm mainly includes liquid embolic agent, balloon or stent assisted coil embolization, Willis covered stent and

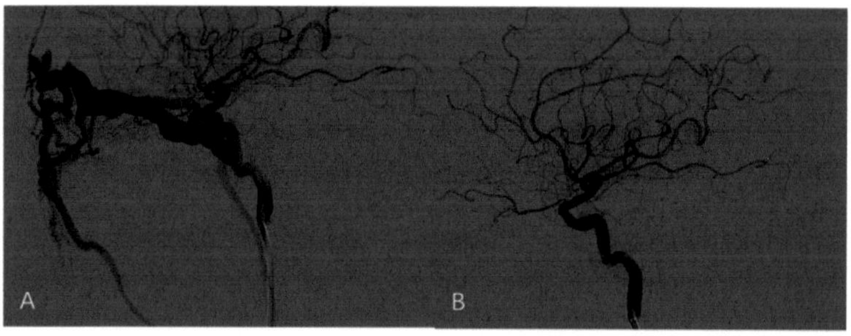

Figure 6.
A 27-year-old woman presented a traumatic CCF treated with detachable balloon. A: Lateral view of the left internal carotid artery angiogram showing a direct CCF of Zipfel's type II with ophthalmic vein reflux. B: Lateral view of the left internal carotid artery angiogram showing complete obliteration of the CCF after detachable balloon embolization.

flow diversion. The Onyx can be injected into the pseudoaneurysm cavity until the aneurysm cavity is completely closed [37]. Balloon or stent can assist coil embolization to prevent the coil from falling out. Willis covered stent can be a curative option and is placed in the parent artery to occlude the neck of pseudoaneurysm. When there are important arterial branches in the lesional area, the application of Willis covered stent may sacrifice the functional branches and cause symptoms of cerebral ischemia. Therefore, its use is limited to the area where no functional branches are found [38].

5.3 Arterial dissection

Coil occlusion of the parent artery is sufficient to prevent subsequent rupture of arterial dissection [39]. This procedure can be performed in the ICA with an open circle of Willis or a vertebral artery with adequate contralateral flow [40]. If the collateral circulation is insufficient, endovascular reconstruction therapy, such as covered stent or flow diversion, may be helpful to preserve the luminal patency and prevent further rupture of the arterial dissection [39].

6. Conclusion

Traumatic injury of internal carotid and vertebral arteries mainly include TCCF, pseudoaneurysm and arterial dissection, which can cause pain, bleeding, edema, diplopia, visual impairment, and death. Cerebral angiography is the gold standard of diagnosis and endovascular treatment is the main method for traumatic neurovascular disease. This chapter helps to understand how endovascular treatments are slowly becoming the norm.

Author details

Huachen Zhang[1], Hanrui Xu[2], Shikai Liang[1] and Xianli Lv[1*]

1 Department of Neurosurgery, Beijing Tsinghua Changgung Hospital, School of Clinical Medicine, Tsinghua University, Beijing, China

2 Department of Neurology, Beijing Tsinghua Changgung Hospital, School of Clinical Medicine, Tsinghua University, Beijing, China

*Address all correspondence to: lvxianli000@163.com

References

[1] Harrigan MR, Hadley MN, Dhall SS, Walters BC, Aarabi B, Gelb DE, et al. Management of vertebral artery injuries following non-penetrating cervical trauma. Neurosurgery. 2013;**72**(Suppl 2):234-243. DOI: 10.1227/NEU.0b013e31827765f5 PMID: 23417194

[2] Higashida RT, Halbach VV, Tsai FY, Norman D, Pribram HF, Mehringer CM, et al. Interventional neurovascular treatment of traumatic carotid and vertebral artery lesions: Results in 234 cases. AJR. American Journal of Roentgenology. 1989;**153**(3):577-582. DOI: 10.2214/ajr.153.3.577 PMID: 2763958

[3] Iorga ER, Costin D. Vascular emergencies in neuro-ophthalmology. Romanian Journal of Ophthalmology. 2020;**64**(4):323-332. DOI: 10.22336/rjo.2020.54 PMID: 33367170; PMCID: PMC7739024

[4] Wang W, Li YD, Li MH, Tan HQ, Gu BX, Wang J, et al. Endovascular treatment of post-traumatic direct carotid-cavernous fistulas: A single-center experience. Journal of Clinical Neuroscience. 2011;**18**(1):24-28. DOI: 10.1016/j.jocn.2010.06.008 PMID: 20888773

[5] Fattahi TT, Brandt MT, Jenkins WS, Steinberg B. Traumatic carotid-cavernous fistula: Pathophysiology and treatment. The Journal of Craniofacial Surgery. 2003;**14**(2):240-246. DOI: 10.1097/00001665-200303000-00020 PMID: 12621297

[6] Liu AF, Li C, Yu W, Lin LM, Qiu HC, Zhang YQ, et al. Dissection-related carotid-cavernous fistula (CCF) following surgical revascularization of chronic internal carotid artery occlusion: A new subtype of CCF and proposed management. Chinese Neurosurgical Journal. 2020;**6**:2. DOI: 10.1186/s41016-019-0180-9 PMID: 32922931; PMCID: PMC7398240

[7] Shih YT, Chen WH, Lee WL, Lee HT, Shen CC, Tsuei YS. Hybrid surgery for symptomatic chronic total occlusion of carotid artery: A technical note. Neurosurgery. 2013;**73**(1 Suppl Operative):E117-E123; discussion ons E123. DOI: 10.1227/NEU.0b013e31827fca6c PMID: 23190641

[8] Barrow DL, Spector RH, Braun IF, Landman JA, Tindall SC, Tindall GT. Classification and treatment of spontaneous carotid-cavernous sinus fistulas. Journal of Neurosurgery. 1985;**62**(2):248-256. DOI: 10.3171/jns.1985.62.2.0248 PMID: 3968564

[9] Zipfel GJ, Shah MN, Refai D, Dacey RG Jr, Derdeyn CP. Cranial dural arteriovenous fistulas: Modification of angiographic classification scales based on new natural history data. Neurosurgical Focus. 2009;**26**(5):E14. DOI: 10.3171/2009.2.FOCUS0928 PMID: 19408992

[10] Zhang H, Zhu K, Wang J, Lv X. The use of a new classification in endovascular treatment of dural arteriovenous fistulas. Neuroscience Informatics. 2022;**2**:100047. DOI: 10.1016/j.neuri.2022.100047

[11] Ringer AJ, Salud L, Tomsick TA. Carotid cavernous fistulas: Anatomy, classification, and treatment. Neurosurgery Clinics of North America. 2005;**16**(2):279-295, viii. DOI: 10.1016/j.nec.2004.08.004 PMID: 15694161

[12] Núñez DB Jr, Torres-León M, Múnera F. Vascular injuries of the

neck and thoracic inlet: Helical CT-angiographic correlation. Radiographics. 2004;**24**(4):1087-1098; discussion 1099-100. DOI: 10.1148/rg.244035035 PMID: 15256630

[13] Saito K, Baskaya MK, Shibuya M, Suzuki Y, Sugita K. False traumatic aneurysm of the dorsal wall of the supraclinoid internal carotid artery--case report. Neurologia Medico-Chirurgica (Tokyo). 1995;**35**(12):886-891. DOI: 10.2176/nmc.35.886 PMID: 8584086

[14] Luo CB, Teng MM, Yen DH, Chang FC, Lirng JF, Chang CY. Endovascular embolization of recurrent traumatic carotid-cavernous fistulas managed previously with detachable balloons. The Journal of Trauma. 2004;**56**(6):1214-1220. DOI: 10.1097/01.ta.0000131213.93205.57 PMID: 15211128

[15] Livshits IM, Berdinov BF, Musa G, Chmutin EG, Levov VA, Chmutin GK, et al. Traumatic intracranial aneurysms (TICA) in children: a description of two clinical cases of successful treatment and review of literature. Childs Nerve System. 24 Aug 2022. DOI: 10.1007/s00381-022-05647-9. Epub ahead of print. PMID: 36002689

[16] Foreman PM, Harrigan MR. Blunt traumatic extracranial cerebrovascular injury and ischemic stroke. Cerebrovascular Diseases Extra. 2017;**7**(1):72-83. DOI: 10.1159/000455391 PMID: 28399527; PMCID: PMC5425764

[17] Dubey A, Sung WS, Chen YY, Amato D, Mujic A, Waites P, et al. Traumatic intracranial aneurysm: A brief review. Journal of Clinical Neuroscience. 2008;**15**(6):609-612. DOI: 10.1016/j.jocn.2007.11.006 PMID: 18395452

[18] Alexander MJ, Smith TP, Tucci DL. Treatment of an iatrogenic petrous carotid artery pseudoaneurysm with a Symbiot covered stent: Technical case report. Neurosurgery. 2002;**50**(3):658-662. DOI: 10.1097/00006123-200203000-00047 PMID: 11841739

[19] Morton RP, Levitt MR, Emerson S, Ghodke BV, Hallam DK, Sekhar LN, et al. Natural history and Management of Blunt Traumatic Pseudoaneurysms of the internal carotid artery: The Harborview algorithm based off a 10-year experience. Annals of Surgery. 2016;**263**(4):821-826. DOI: 10.1097/SLA.0000000000001158 PMID: 25692360

[20] Kansagra AP, Balasetti V, Huang MC. Neurovascular trauma: Diagnosis and therapy. Handbook of Clinical Neurology. 2021;**176**:325-344. DOI: 10.1016/B978-0-444-64034-5.00012-2 PMID: 33272402

[21] Mortazavi MM, Verma K, Tubbs RS, Harrigan M. Pediatric traumatic carotid, vertebral and cerebral artery dissections: A review. Child's Nervous System. 2011;**27**(12):2045-2056. DOI: 10.1007/s00381-011-1409-x PMID: 21318614

[22] Kim SH, Kosnik E, Madden C, Rusin J, Wack D, Bartkowski H. Cerebellar infarction from a traumatic vertebral artery dissection in a child. Pediatric Neurosurgery. 1997;**27**(2):71-77. DOI: 10.1159/000121230 PMID: 9520078

[23] Ito H, Uchida M, Kawaguchi K, Hidaka G, Takasuna H, Goto T, et al. Delayed iatrogenic dissection caused by a carotid stent: A case report. NMC Case Report Journal. 2021;**8**(1):241-245. DOI: 10.2176/nmccrj.cr.2020-0258 PMID: 35079470; PMCID: PMC8769419

[24] Redekop GJ. Extracranial carotid and vertebral artery dissection: A review. The Canadian Journal of Neurological Sciences. 2008;**35**(2):146-152. DOI: 10.1017/s0317167100008556 PMID: 18574926

[25] Wolfe SQ, Mueller-Kronast N, Aziz-Sultan MA, Zauner A,

Bhatia S. Extracranial carotid artery pseudoaneurysm presenting with embolic stroke in a pediatric patient. Case report. Journal of Neurosurgery. Pediatrics. 2008;**1**(3):240-243. DOI: 10.3171/PED/2008/1/3/240 PMID: 18352770

[26] Kieslich M, Fiedler A, Heller C, Kreuz W, Jacobi G. Minor head injury as cause and co-factor in the aetiology of stroke in childhood: A report of eight cases. Journal of Neurology, Neurosurgery, and Psychiatry. 2002;**73**(1):13-16. DOI: 10.1136/jnnp.73.1.13 PMID: 12082038; PMCID: PMC1757298

[27] Debette S, Leys D. Cervical-artery dissections: Predisposing factors, diagnosis, and outcome. Lancet Neurology. 2009;**8**(7):668-678. DOI: 10.1016/S1474-4422(09)70084-5 PMID: 19539238

[28] Steinke W, Rautenberg W, Schwartz A, Hennerici M. Noninvasive monitoring of internal carotid artery dissection. Stroke. 1994;**25**(5):998-1005. DOI: 10.1161/01.str.25.5.998 PMID: 7909394

[29] Xia S, Wang Y, Lv X, Chen C, Hui J, Wu X, Wang Z, Chen H, Ji J. The use of SNAP and T1-weighted VISTA in cervical artery dissection. Interventional Neuroradiology. 2 Mar 2022:15910199221082847. DOI: 10.1177/15910199221082847. Epub ahead of print. PMID: 35234066

[30] Lv XL, Li YX, Liu AH, Lv M, Jiang P, Zhang JB, et al. A complex cavernous sinus dural arteriovenous fistula secondary to covered stent placement for a traumatic carotid artery-cavernous sinus fistula: Case report. Journal of Neurosurgery. 2008;**108**(3):588-590. DOI: 10.3171/JNS/2008/108/3/0588 PMID: 18312107

[31] Brenna CTA, Priola SM, Pasarikovski CR, Ku JC, Daigle P, Gill HS, et al. Surgical sparing and pairing endovascular interventions for carotid-cavernous fistula: Case series and review of the literature. World Neurosurgery. 2020;**140**:18-25. DOI: 10.1016/j.wneu.2020.05.013 PMID: 32437988

[32] Lv X, Jiang C, Li Y, Wu Z. A promising adjuvant to detachable coils for cavernous packing: onyx. Interventional Neuroradiology. 2009;**15**(2):145-152. DOI: 10.1177/159101990901500202 PMID: 20465891; PMCID: PMC3299014

[33] Lv XL. Arteriovenous Malformations of the Brain. NY, USA: NOVA; 2020

[34] Lv X, Li Y, Yang X, Jiang C, Wu Z. Endovascular management of direct carotid-cavernous sinus fistulas. The Neuroradiology Journal. 2012;**25**(1):130-134. DOI: 10.1177/197140091202500117 PMID: 24028886

[35] Wang YL, Ma J, Li YD, Ding PX, Han XW, Wu G. Application of the Willis covered stent for the management of posttraumatic carotid-cavernous fistulas: An initial clinical study. Neurology India. 2012;**60**(2):180-184. DOI: 10.4103/0028-3886.96397 PMID: 22626700

[36] Byrne JV, Beltechi R, Yarnold JA, Birks J, Kamran M. Early experience in the treatment of intra-cranial aneurysms by endovascular flow diversion: A multicentre prospective study. PLoS One. 2010;**5**(9):e12492. DOI: 10.1371/journal.pone.0012492 PMID: 20824070; PMCID: PMC2932685

[37] Jadhav AP, Pryor JC, Nogueira RG. Onyx embolization for the endovascular treatment of infectious and traumatic aneurysms involving the cranial and cerebral vasculature. Journal of NeuroInterventional Surgery. 2013;**5**(6):562-565. DOI: 10.1136/neurintsurg-2012-010460 PMID: 23132531

[38] Lv X, Jiang C, Li Y, Lv M, Zhang J, Wu Z. Intracranial pseudoaneurysms, fusiform aneurysms and carotid-cavernous fistulas. Repair with percutaneous implantation of endovascular covered stents. Interventional Neuroradiology. 2008;**14**(4):435-440. DOI: 10.1177/159101990801400409 PMID: 20557743; PMCID: PMC3313811

[39] Nangarwal B, Bhaisora KS, Khatri D, Sharma A, Singh V, Maurya V, et al. An institutional experience and literature review on iatrogenic major vascular injury in neurosurgery: Proposal of a management algorithm. Neurology India. 2022;**70**(4):1580-1589. DOI: 10.4103/0028-3886.355143 PMID: 36076662

[40] Urasyanandana K, Songsang D, Aurboonyawat T, Chankaew E, Withayasuk P, Churojana A. Treatment outcomes in cerebral artery dissection and literature review. Interventional Neuroradiology. 2018;**24**(3):254-262. DOI: 10.1177/1591019918755692 PMID: 29433365; PMCID: PMC5967189

Chapter 7

Recent Advances in the Development of Biofluid-Based Prognostic Biomarkers of Diffuse Axonal Injury

Vinu V. Gopal, Rinku Raj Mullasseril and Goutam Chandra

Abstract

Even though head injury is a silent pandemic of the century producing immense social and economic impact, predictive models have not been established to develop strategies promoting the development of reliable diagnostic tools and effective therapeutics capable of improving the prognosis. Diffuse axonal injury (DAI) is a type of traumatic brain injury (TBI) that results from a blunt injury to the brain. Discovering biomarkers for DAI have been a matter of debate and research. A number of studies have reported biomarkers that are correlated with severity of TBI but no conclusive and reproducible clinical evidence regarding the same has been put forward till now. Additionally, many DAI biomarkers have limitations so that they cannot be generalized for universal applications. The properties of these biomarkers should be extensively researched along with the development of novel biomarkers to aid important clinical decisions for the benefit of the society. This chapter summarizes the existing biofluid-based biomarkers, critically examines their limitations and highlights the possibilities of a few novel biomolecules as prognostic biomarkers of DAI.

Keywords: diffuse axonal injury, biofluid, neuronal damage, prognosis, rehabilitation

1. Introduction

Central nervous system (CNS) trauma including traumatic brain injury (TBI) is a major cause of long-term injury, disability and death among young adults worldwide [1, 2]. Around 1.6 million individuals suffer from TBI every year in India with 200,000 deaths [3]. In the USA, there were more than 223,000 TBI-related hospitalizations in 2018 and about 166 Americans died from TBI-related injury each day in 2019 [4]. These estimates do not include the many TBIs that are only treated in the emergency department, primary care, urgent care, or those that go untreated [5]. Since the affected individuals are disabled and out of work during the most productive period of their life, these devastating conditions have an enormous physical, mental and economic burden to the country.

IntechOpen

TBI is a heterogeneous neurological condition, ranging from single or repetitive concussion /mild TBI to penetrating head injury, focal contusion, different forms of hematoma (subdural and epidural) and diffuse injury. Depending on the motor, verbal, and eye-opening responses of the affected individuals, the Glasgow coma scale (GCS) was designed to access the disability. The GCS measures the following three functions: Motor response (scores: 6-normal, 5-localized to pain, 4-withdraws to pain, 3-flexion response to pain, 2-extension response to pain, 1-no motor response), Verbal response (scores: 5-normal conversation, 4-oriented conversation, 3-words, but not coherent, 2-no words, only sounds, 1-none), and Eye-opening response (scores: 4-spontaneous, 3-to voice, 2-to pain, 1-none). Based on the GCS score, TBI is classified as mild, moderate, or severe. TBI patients with GCS of 13 to 15 are classified to be mild, which includes the majority of these patients. Patients with a GCS of 9 to 12 are considered to have a moderate TBI, while patients with a GCS below eight are classified as having a severe TBI [6].

The heterogeneous nature of TBI with respect to severity of the injury and comorbidities make patient outcome difficult to predict. While mild TBI or concussion may affect neural cells temporarily, severe TBI is associated with substantial axonal injury and physical damage to the brain, which can result in blood-brain barrier disruption and neuroinflammatory changes [7]. Moderate to severe TBI can usually be visible as structural abnormalities using radiological examinations such as computed tomography (CT) or magnetic resonance imaging (MRI). However, more subtle neural alterations characteristic of mild TBI are not easily detected by these imaging techniques.

Although TBI is an extremely complex condition, there have been many advances in recent years in relation to the diagnosis, monitoring and treatment of the affected patients. Shortcomings in our knowledge of the physiopathology of TBI and the development of reliable predictive models capable of offering an early orientation as to the patient outcome, will improve the diagnostic and therapeutic strategies on an individualized basis. Likewise, we need valid predictive models in severe TBI in order to define efficacy endpoints in the evaluation of new drugs or treatment strategies–since the usual primary endpoints (death and disability) are widely recognized as being inadequate and could explain the discouraging results obtained with certain promising drugs.

2. Pathogenesis of DAI

Diffuse axonal injury (DAI) is a type of TBI that results from a blunt injury to the brain, which happens when the brain rapidly shifts inside the skull as an injury is occurring. It is one of the most common but devastating types of TBI. Neuronal injuries associated with DAI fall into two categories: (i) primary injury, which is directly caused by mechanical forces during the initial insult; and (ii) secondary injury, which is caused as a consequence of primary injury to further tissue and cellular damages.

2.1 Primary brain injuries

Primary brain injuries refer to the sudden and profound injury to the brain that occurs at the time of the motor vehicle accident, gunshot wound, or accidental fall. The immediate impact of different mechanical insults to the brain can cause two types of primary TBI: focal and diffuse brain injuries. Focal TBI generally results from a blow to the head that produces cerebral contusions or hematomas. Epidural hematomas, subdural hematomas, and cerebral contusions are the results of focal brain injuries [8]. In contrast, diffuse lesions (also known as DAI) are seen more commonly in lesions that involve rapid acceleration, deceleration, or rotational forces. DAI accounts for about 70% of TBI cases. The sites that are most prone to DAI are the reticular formation, basal ganglia, superior cerebellar peduncles, limbic fornices, hypothalamus and corpus callosum [8]. Interestingly, both types of injuries may co-exist in patients who suffered from moderate to severe TBI [9].

Brain injuries may occur in one of two ways: closed brain TBI and penetrating TBI. Closed brain TBIs occur when there is a non-penetrating injury to the brain with no break in the skull. A closed brain injury is caused by a rapid forward or backward movement and shaking of the brain inside the bony skull that result in bruising and tearing of brain tissue and blood vessels. In contrast, Penetrating, or open head injuries occur when there is a break in the skull, caused by hitting with a sharp object such as a bullet. These injuries exhibit focal brain damage due to lacerations, compression and concussion forces with evidence of skull fracture and localized contusion (**Figure 1**) at the core of injury site, known as the 'coup' area [10, 11]. Compromised blood supply at the coup area due to epidural, subdural and intracerebral hemorrhages and hematomas might result in necrosis of neuronal and glial cells at confined layers of the brain. Secondary contusion may develop in brain tissues opposite to or surrounding the coup area due to secondary impact when the brain rebounds and strikes the skull [11].

2.2 Secondary brain injuries

Secondary brain injuries refer to the changes that evolve over a period of time after the primary brain injury. The biochemical, cellular and physiological events that occur during primary injury often progress into delayed and prolonged secondary damaging cascade of cellular, chemical, tissue, or blood vessel changes in the brain that contribute to further destruction of brain tissue. Secondary brain injuries can last from hours to days and even weeks and may be caused by impairment or local declines in cerebral blood flow resulting in local edema, hemorrhage, or increased intracranial pressure and even brain herniation. Other types of secondary injury due to TBI include hypercapnia, acidosis, meningitis and brain abscess [12]. Mechanistically, a number of factors contribute to these changes, which include excitotoxicity, loss of cerebral autoregulation, blood-brain barrier compromise, mitochondrial dysfunction, oxidative stress, lipid peroxidation, neuroinflammation, axon degeneration, impaired autophagy and apoptotic cell death (**Figure 1**) [10, 13].

The hallmark feature of DAI is extensive damage of axons predominantly in subcortical and deep white matter tissue, which leads to impairment of axonal transport and degradation of axonal cytoskeleton. The strong tensile forces generated during primary injury by rapid deceleration and acceleration of the brain due to multiple non-contact forces causing shearing and stretching injury in cerebral brain tissues damage neuronal axons, oligodendrocytes and blood vasculature, leading to brain edema and ischemic brain damage [14]. These axonal damages can persist for months after DAI.

The degree of axonal injury and neuronal degeneration determines the severity of TBI. While explosive blast TBI is a result of shock waves instead of inertial forces, it displays the characteristics of a typical DAI. Depending on the severity of the injury, patients may later develop cognitive deficits, behavioral changes and hemiparesis (**Figure 1**).

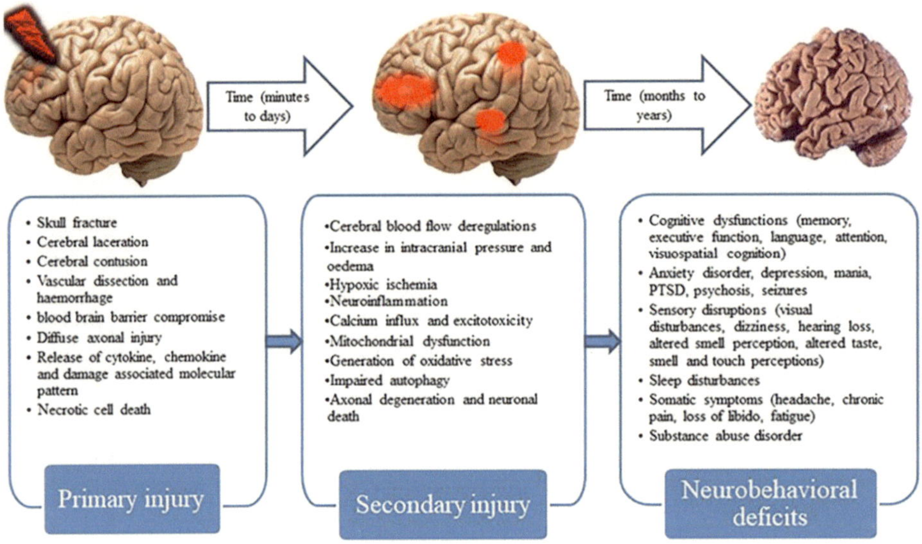

Figure 1.
Schematic representation of the pathogenesis of TBI. TBI *may be divided into* primary *injury and* secondary *injury. Primary* TBI *results from mechanical injury at the time of insult, while secondary injury is caused by the physiologic responses to the initial injury.* Primary *brain injury comprises the direct physical injury to the brain such as compression, deformation, displacement, stretching, shearing, tearing, and crushing of brain which results in damage to vasculature, neural, and glial tissues. Most of the neurological damage from TBI is due to the secondary injury which evolves over the ensuing hours and days after the initial injury or impact. The mechanisms by which TBI trigger neurodegeneration are areas of active research. Previous investigations found roles of excitotoxicity, loss of cerebral autoregulation, blood-brain barrier compromise, mitochondrial dysfunction, oxidative stress, lipid peroxidation, neuroinflammation, axon degeneration, impaired autophagy and apoptotic cell death in the development of neurodegeneration following brain injury. TBI produces both acute and chronic consequences that lead to permanent disabilities that increase long-term mortality and reduced life expectancy. The direct consequences of a single or repetitive TBI can result in various secondary pathological conditions, including seizures, sleep disorders, neurodegenerative diseases, neuroendocrine dysregulation, and psychiatric problems. Changes initiated by TBI can persist for weeks to months or even years after injury and significantly affect quality-of-life of the affected victims.*

3. Need for biofluid-based brain damage biomarkers

While mild TBI or concussion may affect neural cells temporarily, severe TBI is associated with substantial axonal injury and physical damage to the brain, which can result in blood-brain barrier disruption and neuroinflammatory changes [7]. Although, moderate to extensive brain injury may be visible as structural abnormalities using CT scan or MRI, more subtle neural alterations characteristic of mild TBI are not easily detected by these imaging techniques. Moreover, changes due to DAI in the brain are often microscopic and may not be visualized on CT scan or MRI scans.

Mild TBI is highly prevalent in military populations, with many service members suffering from long-term symptoms [15]. It is also very common among road accident victims. The condition results from etiologies of neural contusion and axonal injury, which subsequently results in biochemical, metabolic, and cellular changes that may be responsible for some of the long-term problems observed in patients who develop post-concussion syndrome [16]. Moreover, moderate to severe TBI remains another important public health problem, due to the large percentage of unfavorable outcomes involved such as death and disabling sequelae. The huge treatment costs, associated compensations, disability pensions and years of income from work lost in affected individuals are the major financially devastating turns in the affected families. Therefore, identifying critical markers of neural injury in biofluids of these patients would be crucial for predicting long-term functional outcome and for taking rehabilitation decisions. Encouragingly, significant scientific advances on the TBI biomarker research in the last decade have increased our understanding of the complex and heterogeneous pathophysiological processes associated with this condition. Emerging evidence from multiple research teams suggests that biofluid-based TBI biomarkers may have the potential to diagnose the presence of TBI of different severities, and to predict outcome.

4. Biomarkers for TBI/DAI

A biomarker is defined as a quantifiable biological indicator specific for a given physiological or pathological condition. Based on clinical utility, biomarkers may be categorized as: 1) diagnostic biomarkers, which identify the presence or absence of TBI, 2) prognostic biomarkers, which inform the clinicians about expected outcomes in injured individuals, and 3) predictive biomarkers, which predict response to a specific intervention and can be used to monitor response to therapy. Identification of biological markers of TBI could offer a more precise indication of the extent and severity of TBI, independently of the prior biological substrate and of other circumstances that accompany severe TBI–thereby contributing to homogeneously define different patient categories and risk stratify the head injury. These can also serve to screen and identify patients who may expect an altered or complicated recovery or might develop neurobehavioral deficits during the latter part of their life. Such markers would facilitate

- individualization of the intensity of TBI/DAI
- improve knowledge of the physiopathology of brain damage
- afford essential complementary information for the diagnosis
- predict the outcome of these patients
- timing of patient management
- development of strategies for preventing or minimizing secondary damage
- evaluation of neuroprotective effects of novel biomolecules.

4.1 Which is an ideal biomarker?

An ideal TBI/DAI biomarker should have

- high specificity and sensitivity for the brain tissue

- rapid appearance in accessible biofluids such as cerebrospinal fluid (CSF), plasma and/or whole blood immediately after irreversible brain tissue damage.

- must be elevated in various forms and/or severities of brain damage in the acute phase (3 h to 24 h post-injury).

- must reflect the extent and severity of the damage, as defined by GCS, CT abnormality, in due course of time.

- variations between age and gender groups must be minimal.

- must have low basal biofluid levels in non-injured healthy control population

- should be responsive to therapeutic treatments

- the tools for analysis and immediate detection of the marker must be available and reproducible.

- determination of the marker must be clinically relevant.

The literature given below is a concise description of the principal investigational brain damage biomarkers with a description of the tissues in which they originate, the compartment from which samples were collected, their pathological serum concentrations, and the main prognostic features (**Table 1**).

4.2 Tau protein

Tau protein is an axonal cytoskeleton-stabilizing protein (**Figure 2**) of molecular weight of 30–50 kDa that provides structural elements of the cytoskeleton that are crucial for neuronal protein flow [46, 47]. There are 6 different tau protein isomers, which is phosphorylated at many sites by kinases such as casein kinase II, tau tubulin kinases, glycogen synthase kinase 3β, and cyclin dependent kinase 5 [48–50]. While these are present in a stable, unfolded and monomeric morphology in a healthy brain, tau proteins exist in hyperphosphorylated state in several neurodegenerative diseases including Alzheimer's disease (AD) [46, 51]. Interestingly, TBI has been indicated as a risk factor for later development of AD and other neurodegenerative conditions [52–56] .

Physical trauma causes activation of a number of proteases, which cause release of tau protein fragments in cleaved tau (c-tau) into the blood and CSF [57, 58]. Studies showed that the c-tau levels in CSF increase in the first 24 h after severe TBI [17, 59, 60]. Plasma phosphorylated tau (p-tau) and p-tau/t-tau ratios have been demonstrated to distinguish patients with acute and chronic TBI from healthy controls [18]. Smith and colleagues (1999) have shown deposition of p-tau following TBI [61]. C-tau in CSF is shown to be a predictor of clinical outcomes in severe TBI subjects [60, 62]. Moreover, elevated c-tau could be a chronic manifestation in DAI, since tau is localized to the axons [59]. However, the practical role of this molecule in DAI has not been fully established.

4.3 Amyloid-β (Aβ) protein

Amyloid-β (Aβ) is a 4 kDa extracellular protein derived from amyloid precursor protein (APP), which is cleaved by secretase enzymes [63]. APP is a membrane

Biomarker	Localization	Role in prognosis	Drawbacks	References
Tau/c-tau	Neuronal axons and astrocytes	May predict outcomes after severe TBI	Not fully characterized	[17–19]
Aβ	Extracellular space	Altered levels in CSF	Contradictory findings	[20–22]
MBP	Axonal myelin sheath, oligodendroglial cells	Elevated levels in serum and predict severity and outcome	Limited sensitivity	[23, 24]
CK-BB	astrocytes	May predict outcomes after severe TBI	Low sensitivity and specificity in polytrauma	[25–27]
NSE	Neuron	Elevated serum levels and specific to neuronal tissue than glial cell	Long half-life and are expressed in red blood cells	[28–32]
S100B	Astrocytes	Predict severity and act as adjuvant marker	Reduced specificity; not suitable for children under 2 years	[33, 34]
GFAP	Astrocytes	May predict neurological outcomes	Also expressed by the Leydig cells of the testes	[35–37]
UCH-L1	Neuronal cell body	Increased serum levels in brain damage	Not fully characterized	[38–40]
SBDPs	Axons and presynaptic neuronal endings	May predict neurological outcomes	Not brain specific and difficult to quantify	[41–44]
NfL	Neuronal cytoplasm	Released in response to CNS neuronal damage	Released in response to neurodegeneration and neuroinflammation	[45]

Table 1.
Current and emerging DAI biomarkers.

protein expressed in both CNS (APP 695) and peripheral organs and tissues (APP 751 and APP 770) [64]. APP with 695 amino acids is present as glycosylated receptors on cell surface and is hydrolysed by α-secretase followed by γ-secretase under normal conditions to produce soluble Aβ through non-amyloidogenic pathway [63, 65]. In amyloidogenic pathway, the mutations in APP and components of α-secretase, presinillin 1 (PSEN1) and presinillin 2 (PSEN2) leads to the cleavage by β amyloid cleaving enzyme-1 (BACE1) and γ-secretase to form insoluble Aβ, $A\beta_{1-40}$ and $A\beta_{1-42}$. This amyloidogenic cleavage leads to extracellular accumulation of Aβ plaques, a pathological hallmark in AD [20, 65, 66]. APP plays an important role in cell adhesion processes and thus high concentrations are found at neuronal synaptic junction. Certain type of caspase breaks it down into a series of products which accumulate in cell bodies and axons. There are discordant evidence on the use of this protein as biomarker of TBI. One study of 29 patients with severe TBI revealed low levels of this protein in CSF probably due to reabsorption of the protein in the form of amyloid plaques [21]. As a contradiction to the above, Emmerling et al. (2020) found increasing levels in CSF after trauma and suggested that this could be a result of secondary axonal damage or loss of integrity of the BBB [22]. These contradictory findings, have

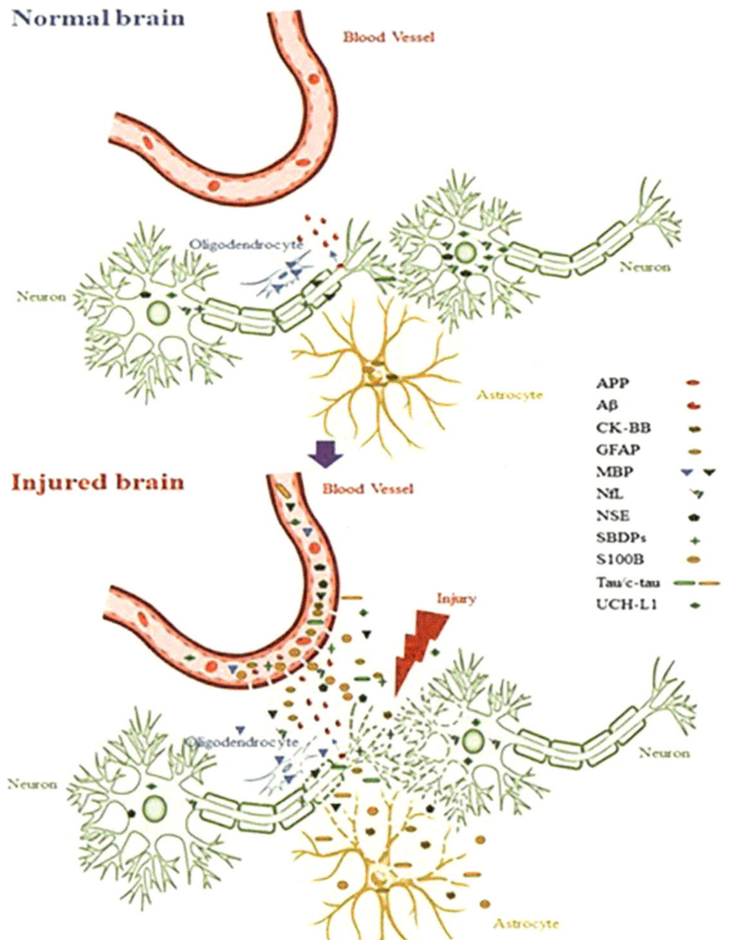

Figure 2.
Origin of biomarkers of DAI. In normal brain, NSE and UCH-L1 are localized in neuronal cytoplasm, while tau/c-tau are restricted mainly to axons and its terminals. Although tau is abundant in the neurons of the CNS, astrocytes express very low levels of this protein and it can be secreted into the brain interstitial fluid. APP is a type I transmembrane protein expressed in many cell types, including neurons. Aβ is derived from APP by enzymatic cleavage and is released to extracellular space. MBP is a constituent of neuronal myelin sheath, which is produced by oligodendrocytes. Spectrins (precursors of SBDPs), specifically βIV-spectrin is concentrated at axon initial segments and nodes of Ranvier. GFAP, CK-BB and S100B are normally present in astrocytes. DAI not only injures pre- and post-synaptic neurons but also damages their synapses, axons, myelin sheaths and neighboring astrocytes, oligodendrocytes, blood microvasculature and even the extracellular matrix network. Damages to specific cells and cellular components during DAI enable release of various molecules contained in those cells into the extracellular space. The released molecules, including those present in extracellular space like Aβ enter the damaged blood vessels and may be detected in the circulation.

caused Aβ-protein to be regarded as a non-reproducible biomarker and its potential role remains unclear requiring further research.

4.4 Myelin basic protein (MBP)

MBP (molecular weight of 18.5 kDa), found in oligodendroglial cells, is a key structural component of the multi-layered myelin sheath covering nerve fibers. The myelin sheath on neuronal axons serves as an insulator to increase the velocity of axonal impulse conduction. Due to the extended length of axonal fiber tracks, axons are particularly vulnerable to physical trauma to the brain. Thus, axonal injury is a common occurrence in both focal as well as diffuse brain trauma and can be found in TBI of all severities [14, 67]. As MBP maintains myelin structure by interacting with the lipids in the myelin membrane [68], axonal injury causes breakdown of the myelin sheath and release of MBP. This myelin-specific protein is also released into the bloodstream in cases of demyelinating diseases such as multiple sclerosis, or degradation by proteases, such as calpain [69, 70].

MBP is found to be elevated in serum after severe TBI in children [23, 24] and after mild TBI in adults [24]. Even though, it takes around 1–2 days to appear in the serum after TBI, the peak levels of MBP can persist for up to 2 weeks and can be a specific indicator for future intracranial hemorrhage [71]. However, as per present literature there is contradicting evidence for its role in TBI/DAI [72–74]. There was no difference in initial levels of serum MBP in a pediatric population with mild TBI when compared with controls, but there was a significant difference in the peak MBP levels between patients and controls [72]. MBP is also expressed on the myelin of peripheral nerves and its transcripts are present in the bone marrow and immune system and therefore it is not specific to the CNS. Even though serum levels are correlated with patient severity and outcome [71, 75] it has limited sensitivity as a marker for predicting severity of TBI [76].

4.5 Cerebral creatine kinase (CK) isoenzyme

CK isoenzymes are of three types: CK-1 (also known as CK-BB) is predominantly expressed in brain, lung, thyroid and prostate glands, gastrointestinal tract, urinary bladder, uterus and placenta. CK-2 (CK-MB) and CK-3 (CK-MM) are expressed in cardiac and skeletal muscles [77]. Brain tissue-specific CK-1 (CK-BB), with a molecular weight of 40–53 kDa, is found in astrocytes [25, 26]. A peak in serum cerebral CK concentration is observed in the first few hours after severe TBI and then gradually decrease and the marker remains high for days [78–81]. In polytrauma, it remains persistently high without an initial dip [82, 83] . Its levels have been shown to rise significantly in CSF following hypoxic brain injury in cardiac arrest, which suggests that CK-BB release may be secondary to cerebral hypoperfusion due to systemic trauma [84]. The major limiting factor is that it has low sensitivity and specificity especially in cases of polytrauma [27, 85].

4.6 Neuron-specific enolase (NSE)

NSE, also known as γ -enolase or enolase 2, is a glycolytic enzyme with a molecular weight of 78 kDa and a half-life of 48 h. It exists as a homodimer (γ–γ) in mature neurons and neuroendocrine cells. The normal concentration of NSE in blood is <10 ng/ml. NSE elevations in blood compartment has been documented in severe as well as mild TBI [28–31, 86]. Experimental models of trauma have correlated serum NSE to the severity of damage in TBI [87]. Major limitation of using NSE as specific biomarker for TBI is that it is also abundantly expressed in red blood cells [88]. Moreover, increased levels of NSE was also recorded previously in the serum of patients following non-traumatic brain damage such as ischemic events, intracerebral hemorrhage, cardiopulmonary resuscitation, secondary cerebral hypoxia etc. [89]. Some studies had correlated the biomarker to the development of DAI, though its behavior has not been clearly established in prospective trials.

NSE was initially suggested to be a very promising TBI severity marker due to its specificity to neuronal tissue than of glial cells. However, the results published till date has been contradictory on its role in predicting prognosis of patients with severe TBI. Long half-life is a major limiting factor for its use in trauma setting. Also, extracranial origin of NSE was demonstrated in hemorrhagic shock, long bone fracture, hemolysis, heart surgery, ischemia–reperfusion injury and malignant lung tumors making it a poor marker for TBI [90–94].

4.7 Glial fibrillary acidic protein (GFAP)

GFAP is a monomeric intermediate filament protein (molecular weight 52 kDa), present in the cytoskeleton of astrocytes in the brain. An increase in blood level of this biomarker suggests injury to the astrocytes and the BBB. Plasma concentrations >0.033 μg/l are regarded as pathological. Missler et al. (2002) were the first to propose the possible use of GFAP as an identifier of brain damage in serial serum measurements [95]. Later studies also confirmed that the serum concentration of this protein is not affected by extracranial injuries thus making it an effective biomarker for predicting poor outcome in the acute phase of severe TBI as well as for advocating the need for urgent neurosurgical procedures [41, 96]. GFAP (52 kDa) or its breakdown products (44–38 kDa) are released from injured brain tissue into biofluids such as CSF and enter the bloodstream after crossing the BBB with an early plasma peak (within 3 to 34 h) following brain injury [97, 98]. The blood levels then decrease gradually over the first week, starting from third day of injury.

Previous studies demonstrated that GFAP levels show an unfavorable outcome in patients with moderate or severe TBI [41, 96, 99, 100]. However, this may not be the case in patients with mild TBI due to the contamination from other sources [101–103]. However, Serum GFAP levels were also significantly higher in patients who died or had an unfavorable outcome [104]. Moreover, GFAP levels have correctly predicted neurological outcome at 6 months [35, 36, 104]. Furthermore, serum GFAP measured on day 1 of injury in pediatric TBI cases significantly correlated with functional outcomes at 6 months [105]. Thus, GFAP can be considered as an ideal biomarker of brain damage when combined with clinical variables though multicenter studies are needed for further validation.

4.8 S100-calcium binding protein B (S100B)

S100B, the most widely studied brain damage biomarker, is a low molecular weight (11 kDa) calcium binding protein of astroglial origin [33]. The homodimeric beta-subtype of S100 proteins (S100B) is synthesized in astrocytes of the CNS and in Schwann cells of the peripheral nerves, where it regulates intracellular calcium levels [106–108]. S100B localizes to the nucleus and cytoplasm associating with endomembranes, the centrosomes, microtubules and type III intermediate filaments [109]. The protein is naturally secreted by astrocytes into the extracellular space. Low amounts of S100B can cross the BBB and enter the microvasculature. Elevated levels of S100B in the serum were observed in TBI patients as well as in patients suffering from neurodegenerative diseases [110]. The serum levels of the protein have been associated with clinical severity, radiological severity, and an unfavorable outcome [111–114] .

The biological function of this protein has not been fully established till date, though it is known to participate in neurogenesis, astrocytosis and axonal elongation. However, the molecule can also be produced and found outside the CNS, e.g., in kidney epithelial cells, ependymocytes, chondrocytes, adipocytes, melanocytes, Langerhans cells, dendritic cells, certain lymphocyte subpopulations, skeletal myofibers, myoblasts and muscle satellite cells [109]. Metabolism takes place in the kidneys, followed by excretion in urine, with an approximate half-life of 30–113 min, and is not affected by hemolytic phenomena [115]. Its role in urine level also needs further validated study. Since S100B can also be released from adipose tissue and cardiac/skeletal muscles, its levels are also elevated in orthopedic trauma without head injury [116]. Despite these confounders, S100B is actually a sensitive TBI biomarker for predicting CT abnormality and post-concussive syndrome development [117–119]. A number of previous studies have shown that S100B can actually differentiate between mild and severe TBI [120, 121].

The maximum serum concentration of S100B is reached 20 min after brain damage. The normal upper limit for this protein in relation to the detection of intracranial damage was defined as 0.1 μg/l based on a multicenter study in patients with mild TBI [122]. The measurement of S100B-protein can be influenced by patient age and gender in CSF samples but not in serum samples thus making it a practically feasible biomarker.

Some studies have determined its usefulness as a predictor of mortality, establishing orientative serum cut-off points for predicting a course leading to death or an unfavorable outcome [123–125]. On the other hand, S100B level has been correlated to the presence of secondary lesions, the extent of diffuse brain damage, and to modifications in intracranial pressure following different release patterns [126, 127]. S100B levels can also detect brain death development or mortality after severe TBI [128, 129]. Interestingly, serum levels of S100B > 0.7 ng/mL were reported to correlate with 100% mortality [130].

Another possible application of this protein refers to its time course according to the severity of the patient condition. A number of studies have documented persistently elevated serum levels in patients in those with poor GCS, while the plasma levels have been seen to decrease after 36 h among survivors [82, 131–133]. On the other hand, S100B protein has been suggested as a tool for monitoring management efficacy [134, 135], since it has been seen that the blood concentrations of the protein decrease after effective neurosurgical treatment thus making its role more relevant. A high level of S100B during the initial TBI can predict a poor outcome, especially if it is accompanied by a second increase in levels of serum S100B that occurs during the subacute phase [131, 136]. This second peak during the subacute phase may be due to secondary injury to the astroglial cells exhibiting excitotoxicity and neuroinflammation. In addition, elevation in serum levels of S100B and GFAP in TBI patients has been correlated with unfavorable neurological outcomes [137–139]. On the other hand, an initial lower level of S100B and the lack of second peak might suggest the occurrence of a mild TBI and a good functional recovery [140, 141].

A previous study demonstrated the sensitivity of S100B to predict significant intracranial pathology up to 100% but with specificity of only 28%.Moreover, in pediatric population (specifically for children under the age of 2 years), S100B is not a useful marker due to high normal levels in this group [32, 142]. Thus, S100B may be suggested to be used as an adjuvant marker in patients with TBI, but its diagnostic value is still controversial [76].

5. Limitations of the existing biomarkers

Doctors in the acute hospital settings primarily rely on the patient's neurological examinations and radiologic imaging to characterize TBI/DAI diagnosis. Depending on the severity of the initial insult, different imaging modalities such as CT scan and MRI are used to obtain the necessary information for patient care and prognosis. However, CT scans, used for assessing cerebrovascular integrity or for determining gross anatomical changes induced to the brain, have low sensitivity to diffuse brain damage, and confers exposure to radiation [143]. In contrast, while MRI can provide information on the extent of diffuse injuries, yet its widespread application is restricted by prohibitive cost, limited availability of MRI in many hospitals, and practical difficulty of performing it in physiologically unstable TBI patients [143]. Thus, diagnostic and prognostic tools for risk stratification of TBI patients are very limited in the early stages after injury.

To fill this gap, research in the field of biofluid-based TBI biomarkers has increased exponentially over the last three decades [116]. Extensive research on fluid biomarkers have demonstrated that a number of brain-specific proteins, as illustrated above, have potential for acting as biomarkers of TBI. These biomolecules are released into the CSF and/or blood, after brain injury due to damage of neural cells [28, 144–146]. Additionally, neuroimmune activation might have the potential to be novel diagnostic and/or prognostic marker of TBI. A few of these molecules, like S100B have shown promise to be clinically used as biomarkers of TBI [145]. However, this has been disputed in recent studies [147] and till now, there are no rapid, definitive diagnostic blood tests for TBI.

Despite its high sensitivity and negative predictive value, S100B protein is not a specific marker of the CNS damage. Polytraumatized patients without TBI can present S100B protein elevations in blood, though the concentrations return to normal within 6 h after trauma. Patients with brain damage and associated extracranial injuries (hypotension, hypothermia, coagulopathy, inotropic drugs, sedatives, corticosteroids, etc.) can alter the early assessment of S100B protein. Therefore, early determination of this protein is to be avoided in patients with extracranial injuries associated with TBI making it's role dismal probably in trauma care even though the above features of an ideal biomarker are met.

5.1 Difficulty with interpretation

CNS is very complex and can present a range of different lesions, which in turn can affect different target cells with variable degrees of severity. Brain damage markers must establish differentiations with respect to other alterations. Furthermore, the existence of the blood–brain barrier conditions the structural characteristics of these biomarkers, which must be able to cross the mentioned barrier in order to reach the bloodstream. Biomarkers are dynamic elements that experience changes in response to different inflammatory states, tissue necrosis etc. So serial measurements rather than isolated or point determinations are thus required.

5.2 Controversy

As direct sampling of the damaged brain tissue is not practically feasible there is some controversy regarding the type of biological fluid that should be analyzed. CSF compartment is located closer to the damage site, but frequent collection of CSF samples is unethical. As a result, most biomarkers are studied in peripheral blood as the process is simple, accessible and reproducible. Thus, estimation of blood biomarkers will be the most appropriate option for performing simple and minimally invasive serial measurements. Still more easy will be to estimate biomarkers in fluids that serve as vehicles for their clearance, for example urine.

6. Newly discovered biomarkers of interest.

6.1 Ubiquitin carboxy-terminal hydrolase L1 (UCH-L1)

UCH-L1 mainly resides in the cytoplasm of neuronal cell body representing approximately 5% of all the soluble brain proteins. It is implicated in the elimination of degraded and denatured proteins following oxidative phenomena [148]. Proteomics data first implicate UCH-L1 as promising TBI biomarker candidate [149, 150]. Later studies point to it as a promising brain damage biomarker, since there are data indicating that it can predict the presence of lesions on the CT scan, the need for neurosurgery, and the outcome of patients with TBI [151–153].

UCH-L1 can be detected in blood, with early increases in its serum concentration following brain injury [151]. The protein level in the blood is shown to be elevated both in mild and severe cases of TBI [100, 154]. Mondello et al. (2012) have obtained interesting results regarding its possible capacity to distinguish between focal and diffuse brain damage [155]. Additionally, it has been suggested that UCH-L1 together with GFAP form the foundation of a biomarker panel representing the two dominant cell types (neuron and astrocytes) in the brain [38]. Interestingly, serum levels of both of these proteins are elevated in professional breacher trainees who were exposed to repeated explosive discharges as well as athletes who experienced concussions [39, 40]. Further investigations are needed to evaluate the properties of this protein as a promising biomarker of DAI.

7. Spectrin degradation products (SBDPs)

Spectrin is a cytoskeletal protein that lines the intracellular side of the plasma membrane forming a scaffold, which maintains plasma membrane integrity and cytoskeletal structure [156]. It is a heterodimeric protein, composed of two α and two β chains, and contains 106 contiguous amino acid sequence motifs called "spectrin repeats", which are essential to diverse cell functions such as cell adhesion, cell spreading, and the cell cycle [156].

Necrotic and apoptotic cell death during primary and secondary brain injury respectively, cause overactivation of cysteine proteases, such as calpain and caspase-3. These proteases cleave components of the axonal cytoskeleton [157] including spectrin resulting in generation of SBDPs with characteristic molecular weights [26, 158]. The presence of degradation products of spectrin has been described in the CNS in axons and presynaptic neuronal endings [23, 44, 159, 160]. However, SBDPs are not brain specific and its increased serum levels may reflect multiorgan damage in trauma [42, 161]. Moreover, accurate quantification of brain-derived SBDPs in blood is difficult since some proteins found in erythrocytes are similar to those found in the neuronal cytoskeleton [162], thus reducing the diagnostic value of SBDPs.

8. Neurofilament light chain (NfL)

Neurofilaments, consisting of three chains, light (L), medium (M) and heavy (H), make up part of the axonal cytoskeleton. NfL is 68 kDa subunit of the neurofilaments located on the neuronal cytoplasm which is released in response to CNS neuronal damage due to neuroinflammation, neurodegeneration, and/or traumatic or vascular injury [163, 164]. Following axon damage, the influx of calcium alters the phosphorylation state of NfL and subsequent proteolysis. As a result, there is loss of cytoskeletal structure and NfL is released into both CSF and the bloodstream [165]. A number of investigational studies have underscored the role of NfL as biomarker of axon damage [45, 166, 167]. Serum NfL has been shown to distinguish patients with mild, moderate or severe TBI for months and even years after injury [168]. However, serum detection of NfH is considered a better biomarker candidate [169].

9. Conclusions

Since all brain damage biomarkers have some limitation precluding their universal application in the management of severe TBI/DAI, they do not yet form part of routine clinical practice. Some markers, such as NSE and S100B protein, have shown good correlations to clinical severity, the extent of brain damage, response to treatment, and patient outcome. However, the limitations associated with the clinical yield of the molecule or invasiveness of the technique required to obtain the sample have not allowed their generalized use in this patient population.

On the other hand, further studies are needed to understand the role of these proteins in the physiology of the CNS and in the physiopathology of severe TBI/DAI, as well as to clarify the usefulness of those biomarkers that appear to be promising in this field. In this respect, mention must be made of nervous tissue-specific GFAP, as well as of other biomarkers that are currently the focus of interest, such as ubiquitin carboxy-terminal hydrolase L1, the light neurofilaments and spectrin degradation products.

Since these molecules offer isolated information on some of the many elements implicated in the physiopathology of TBI/DAI, we believe that the best strategy is to analyze them in combination. Rather than seeking a biomarker exclusive for brain damage, this approach would allow us to define a panel of biomarkers which jointly – and considering the characteristics inherent to each of them–could offer information referred to severity, the potential benefits of management, and the evolutive course of patients following severe TBI. Only in this way can we hope to complement the traditional methods with a tool that is simple, non-invasive, reproducible and extraordinarily useful for addressing and managing severe TBI/DAI. Moreover, since TBI/DAI is quite complex heterogeneous conditions, it might be clinically justified to use multi-modal biomarkers to evaluate the status of full clinical endophenotypes by combining a panel of biofluid-based and physiologic biomarkers coupled with advanced neuroimaging that are appropriately obtained at multiple time points during the time course of TBI/DAI.

Conflicts of interest

The authors declare that they have no conflicts of interest.

Financial support

RRM is a senior research fellow of Indian Council of Medical Research (ICMR), Government of India. GC is supported by The Ramalingaswami fellowship from the Department of Biotechnology, and grants from the Department of Health Research and ICMR, Government of India.

Author details

Vinu V. Gopal[1*], Rinku Raj Mullasseril[2] and Goutam Chandra[2*]

1 Department of Neurosurgery, Government Medical College, Kottayam, Kerala, India

2 Center for Development and Aging Research, Inter-University Center for Biomedical Research and Super Specialty Hospital, Kottayam, Kerala, India

*Address all correspondence to: vinu.acme5.kottayam@gmail.com; gchandra@iucbr.ac.in

References

[1] Werner C, Engelhard K. Pathophysiology of traumatic brain injury. British Journal of Anaesthesia. 2007;**99**:4-9. DOI: 10.1093/BJA/AEM131

[2] Hoffman SW, Harrison C. The interaction between psychological health and traumatic brain injury: A neuroscience perspective. The Clinical Neuropsychologist. 2009;**23**:1400-1415. DOI: 10.1080/13854040903369433

[3] Kalra S, Banderwal R, Arora K, Kumar S, Singh G, Chawla PA, et al. An update on pathophysiology and treatment of sports-mediated brain injury. Environmental Science and Pollution Research International. 2022;**29**:16786-16798. DOI: 10.1007/S11356-021-18391-5

[4] Center for Disease Control. Injury Prevention and Control: Traumatic Brain Injury – Concussion. n.d. Available from: https://www.google.com/search?q=CDC%2C+2022.+Injury+Prevention+and+Control%3A+Traumatic+Brain+Injury+Center+for+Disease+Control+(CDC)+and+Prevention.&rlz=1C1YQLS_enIN892IN892&oq=CDC%2C+2022.+Injury+Prevention+and+Control%3A+Traumatic+Brain+Injury+Center+f [Accessed: February 9, 2022]

[5] Bell JM, Breiding MJ, DePadilla L. CDC's efforts to improve traumatic brain injury surveillance. Journal of Safety Research. 2017;**62**:253-256. DOI: 10.1016/J.JSR.2017.04.002

[6] Mesfin FB, Gupta N, Shapshak AH, Taylor RS. Diffuse axonal injury. Encycl. Neurological Sciences. 2021:10-12. DOI: 10.1016/b0-12-226870-9/00726-7

[7] Wilson L, Stewart W, Dams-O'Connor K, Diaz-Arrastia R, Horton L, Menon DK, et al. The chronic and evolving neurological consequences of traumatic brain injury. Lancet Neurology. 2017;**16**:813-825. DOI: 10.1016/S1474-4422(17)30279-X

[8] Huffman JC, Brennan MM, Smith FA, Stern TA. 19 – Patients with neurologic conditions I. seizure disorders (including nonepileptic seizures), cerebrovascular disease, and traumatic brain injury. Massachusetts General Hospital Handbook of General Hospital Psychiatry, Elsevier. 2010:237-253. DOI: 10.1016/B978-1-4377-1927-7.00019-4

[9] Skandsen T, Kvistad KA, Solheim O, Strand IH, Folvik M, Anne V. Prevalence and impact of diffuse axonal injury in patients with moderate and severe head injury: A cohort study of early magnetic resonance imaging findings and 1-year outcome: Clinical article. Journal of Neurosurgery. 2010;**113**:556-563. DOI: 10.3171/2009.9.JNS09626

[10] Ng SY, Lee AYW. Traumatic brain injuries: Pathophysiology and potential therapeutic targets. Frontiers in Cellular Neuroscience. 2019;**13**:528. DOI: 10.3389/FNCEL.2019.00528

[11] Schmidt OI, Morganti-Kossmann MC, Heyde CE, Perez D, Yatsiv I, Shohami E, et al. Tumor necrosis factor-mediated inhibition of interleukin-18 in the brain: A clinical and experimental study in head-injured patients and in a murine model of closed head injury. Journal of Neuroinflammation. 2004;**1**:1-6. DOI: 10.1186/1742-2094-1-13

[12] Ganju A. Intensive care in neurosurgery. The Journal of Trauma and Acute Care Surgery. 2003;**54**:798. DOI: 10.1097/01.ta.0000058928.27063.6e

[13] Ray SK, Dixon CE, Banik NL. Molecular mechanisms in the pathogenesis of traumatic brain injury. Histology and Histopathology. 2002;**17**:1137-1152. DOI: 10.14670/HH-17.1137

[14] Smith DH, Meaney DF, Shull WH. Diffuse axonal injury in head trauma. The Journal of Head Trauma Rehabilitation. 2003;**18**:307-316. DOI: 10.1097/00001199-200307000-00003

[15] Philippi CL, Velez CS, Wade BSC, Drennon AM, Cooper DB, Kennedy JE, et al. Distinct patterns of resting-state connectivity in U.S. service members with mild traumatic brain injury versus posttraumatic stress disorder. Brain Imaging and Behavior. 2021;**15**:2616-2626. DOI: 10.1007/S11682-021-00464-1

[16] Zhang J, Puvenna V, Janigro D. Biomarkers of traumatic brain injury and their relationship to pathology. In: Translational Research in Traumatic Brain Injury. Boca Raton (FL): CRC Press; 2016. pp. 263-276. DOI: 10.1201/b18959-17

[17] Chatfield DA, Zemlan FP, Day DJ, Menon DK. Discordant temporal patterns of S100beta and cleaved tau protein elevation after head injury: A pilot study. British Journal of Neurosurgery. 2002;**16**:471-476. DOI: 10.1080/02688690210000030285

[18] Rubenstein R, Chang B, Yue JK, Chiu A, Winkler EA, Puccio AM, et al. Comparing plasma phospho tau, total tau, and phospho tau-total tau ratio as acute and chronic traumatic brain injury biomarkers. JAMA Neurology. 2017;**74**:1063-1072. DOI: 10.1001/JAMANEUROL.2017.0655

[19] Liliang PC, Liang CL, Lu K, Wang KW, Weng HC, Hsieh CH, et al. Relationship between injury severity and serum tau protein levels in traumatic brain injured rats. Resuscitation. 2010;**81**:1205-1208. DOI: 10.1016/J.RESUSCITATION.2010.05.016

[20] Du X, Wang X, Geng M. Alzheimer's disease hypothesis and related therapies. Translational Neurodegeneration. 2018;7:1-7. DOI: 10.1186/s40035-018-0107-y

[21] Franz G, Beer R, Kampfl A, Engelhardt K, Schmutzhard E, Ulmer H, et al. Amyloid beta 1-42 and tau in cerebrospinal fluid after severe traumatic brain injury. Neurology. 2003;**60**:1457-1461. DOI: 10.1212/01.WNL.0000063313.57292.00

[22] Emmerling MR, Morganti-Kossmann MC, Kossmann T, Stahel PF, Watson MD, Evans LM, et al. Traumatic brain injury elevates the Alzheimer's amyloid peptide Aβ42 in human CSF. A possible role for nerve cell injury. Annals of the New York Academy of Sciences. 2000;**903**:118-122. DOI: 10.1111/J.1749-6632.2000.TB06357.X

[23] Ringger NC, O'Steen BE, Brabham JG, Silver X, Pineda J, Wang KKW, et al. A novel marker for traumatic brain injury: CSF alphaII-spectrin breakdown product levels. Journal of Neurotrauma. 2004;**21**:1443-1456. DOI: 10.1089/NEU.2004.21.1443

[24] Zhang Z, Moghieb A, Wang KKW. Neuro-proteomics and neuro-systems biology in the quest of TBI biomarker discovery. In: Biomarkers of the Brain Injury and Neurological Disorders. Boca Raton (FL): CRC Press; 2014. pp. 21-59. DOI: 10.1201/b17644-7

[25] Thompson RJ, Kynoch PAM, Sarjant J. Immunohistochemical localization of creatine kinase-BB isoenzyme to astrocytes in human brain.

Brain Research. 1980;**201**:423-426. DOI: 10.1016/0006-8993(80)91046-X

[26] Toman E, Harrisson S, Belli T. Biomarkers in traumatic brain injury: A review. Journal of the Royal Army Medical Corps. 2016;**162**:103-108. DOI: 10.1136/JRAMC-2015-000517

[27] Ingebrigtsen T, Romner B. Biochemical serum markers of traumatic brain injury. The Journal of Trauma. 2002;**52**:798-808. DOI: 10.1097/00005373-200204000-00038

[28] Buonora JE, Yarnell AM, Lazarus RC, Mousseau M, Latour LL, Rizoli SB, et al. Multivariate analysis of traumatic brain injury: Development of an assessment score. Frontiers in Neurology. 2015;**6**:68. DOI: 10.3389/FNEUR.2015.00068

[29] Böhmer AE, Oses JP, Schmidt AP, Perón CS, Krebs CL, Oppitz PP, et al. Neuron-specific enolase, S100B, and glial fibrillary acidic protein levels as outcome predictors in patients with severe traumatic brain injury. Neurosurgery. 2011;**68**:1624-1630. DOI: 10.1227/NEU.0B013E318214A81F

[30] Stein DM, Kufera JA, Lindell A, Murdock KR, Menaker J, Bochicchio GV, et al. Association of CSF biomarkers and secondary insults following severe traumatic brain injury. Neurocritical Care. 2011;**14**:200-207. DOI: 10.1007/S12028-010-9496-1

[31] Topolovec-Vranic J, Pollmann-Mudryj MA, Ouchterlony D, Klein D, Spence J, Romaschin A, et al. The value of serum biomarkers in prediction models of outcome after mild traumatic brain injury. The Journal of Trauma. 2011;**71**:S478-S486. DOI: 10.1097/TA.0B013E318232FA70

[32] Berger RP, Dulani T, Adelson PD, Leventhal JM, Richichi R, Kochanek PM. Identification of inflicted traumatic brain injury in well-appearing infants using serum and cerebrospinal markers: A possible screening tool. Pediatrics. 2006;**117**:325-332. DOI: 10.1542/PEDS.2005-0711

[33] Gonçalves CA, Concli Leite M, Nardin P. Biological and methodological features of the measurement of S100B, a putative marker of brain injury. Clinical Biochemistry. 2008;**41**:755-763. DOI: 10.1016/J.CLINBIOCHEM.2008.04.003

[34] Calcagnile O, Undén L, Undén J. Clinical validation of S100B use in management of mild head injury. BMC Emergency Medicine. 2012;**12**:1-6. DOI: 10.1186/1471-227X-12-13

[35] Czeiter E, Mondello S, Kovacs N, Sandor J, Gabrielli A, Schmid K, et al. Brain injury biomarkers may improve the predictive power of the IMPACT outcome calculator. Journal of Neurotrauma. 2012;**29**:1770. DOI: 10.1089/NEU.2011.2127

[36] Mondello S, Kobeissy F, Vestri A, Hayes RL, Kochanek PM, Berger RP. Serum concentrations of ubiquitin C-terminal hydrolase-L1 and glial fibrillary acidic protein after pediatric traumatic brain injury. Scientific Reports. 2016;**6**:1-8. DOI: 10.1038/SREP28203

[37] Davidoff MS, Middendorff R, Köfüncü E, Müller D, Ježek D, Holstein AF. Leydig cells of the human testis possess astrocyte and oligodendrocyte marker molecules. Acta Histochemica. 2002;**104**:39-49. DOI: 10.1078/0065-1281-00630

[38] Welch RD, Ayaz SI, Lewis LM, Unden J, Chen JY, Mika VH, et al. Ability of serum glial fibrillary acidic protein, ubiquitin C-terminal hydrolase-L1, and S100B to differentiate normal and

abnormal head computed tomography findings in patients with suspected mild or moderate traumatic brain injury. Journal of Neurotrauma. 2016;**33**:203. DOI: 10.1089/NEU.2015.4149

[39] Tate CM, Wang KKW, Eonta S, Zhang Y, Carr W, Tortella FC, et al. Serum brain biomarker level, neurocognitive performance, and self-reported symptom changes in soldiers repeatedly exposed to low-level blast: A breacher pilot study. Journal of Neurotrauma. 2013;**30**:1620-1630. DOI: 10.1089/NEU.2012.2683

[40] Puvenna V, Brennan C, Shaw G, Yang C, Marchi N, Bazarian JJ, et al. Significance of ubiquitin carboxy-terminal hydrolase L1 elevations in athletes after sub-concussive head hits. PLoS One. 2014;**9**:e96296. DOI: 10.1371/JOURNAL.PONE.0096296

[41] Zoltewicz JS, Mondello S, Yang B, Newsom KJ, Kobeissy F, Yao C, et al. Biomarkers track damage after graded injury severity in a rat model of penetrating brain injury. Journal of Neurotrauma. 2013;**30**:1161-1169. DOI: 10.1089/NEU.2012.2762

[42] Yan X-X, Jeromin A. Spectrin breakdown products (SBDPs) as potential biomarkers for neurodegenerative diseases. Current Translational Geriatrics and Experimental Gerontology Reports. 2012;**1**:85-93. DOI: 10.1007/s13670-012-0009-2

[43] Mondello S, Robicsek SA, Gabrielli A, Brophy GM, Papa L, Tepas J, et al. αII-Spectrin breakdown products (SBDPs): Diagnosis and outcome in severe traumatic brain injury patients. Journal of Neurotrauma. 2010;**27**:1203. DOI: 10.1089/NEU.2010.1278

[44] Pineda JA, Lewis SB, Valadka AB, Papa L, Hannay HJ, Heaton SC, et al. Clinical significance of alphaII-spectrin breakdown products in cerebrospinal fluid after severe traumatic brain injury. Journal of Neurotrauma. 2007;**24**:354-366. DOI: 10.1089/NEU.2006.003789

[45] Sass D, Guedes VA, Smith EG, Vorn R, Devoto C, Edwards KA, et al. Sex differences in behavioral symptoms and the levels of circulating GFAP, tau, and NfL in patients with traumatic brain injury. Frontiers in Pharmacology. 2021;**12**:3367. DOI: 10.3389/FPHAR.2021.746491

[46] Khatoon S, Grundke-Iqbal I, Iqbal K. Levels of normal and abnormally phosphorylated tau in different cellular and regional compartments of Alzheimer disease and control brains. FEBS Letters. 1994;**351**:80-84. DOI: 10.1016/0014-5793(94)00829-9

[47] Mandelkow EM, Mandelkow E. Biochemistry and cell biology of tau protein in neurofibrillary degeneration. Cold Spring Harbor Perspectives in Medicine. 2012;**2**:1-25. DOI: 10.1101/CSHPERSPECT.A006247

[48] Duan Y, Dong S, Gu F, Hu Y, Zhao Z. Advances in the pathogenesis of Alzheimer's disease: Focusing on tau-mediated neurodegeneration. Translational Neurodegeneration. 2012;**1**:24. DOI: 10.1186/2047-9158-1-24

[49] Yang Z, Wang P, Morgan D, Lin D, Pan J, Lin F, et al. Temporal MRI characterization, neurobiochemical and neurobehavioral changes in a mouse repetitive concussive head injury model. Scientific Reports 2015;5(1):1-15. doi:10.1038/srep11178

[50] Rubenstein R, Chang B, Davies P, Wagner AK, Robertson CS, Wang KKW. A novel, ultrasensitive assay for tau: Potential for assessing traumatic brain

injury in tissues and biofluids. Journal of Neurotrauma. 2015;**32**:342. DOI: 10.1089/NEU.2014.3548

[51] Mandelkow EM, Mandelkow E. Biochemistry and cell biology of tau protein in neurofibrillary degeneration. Cold Spring Harbor Perspectives in Biology. 2011;**3**:1-25. DOI: 10.1101/cshperspect.a006247

[52] Iqbal K, Grundke-Iqbal I. Ubiquitination and abnormal phosphorylation of paired helical filaments in Alzheimer's disease. Molecular Neurobiology. 1991;**5**:399-410. DOI: 10.1007/BF02935561

[53] Moretti L, Cristofori I, Weaver SM, Chau A, Portelli JN, Grafman J. Cognitive decline in older adults with a history of traumatic brain injury. Lancet Neurology. 2012;**11**:1103-1112. DOI: 10.1016/S1474-4422(12)70226-0

[54] Sivanandam TM, Thakur MK. Traumatic brain injury: A risk factor for Alzheimer's disease. Neuroscience and Biobehavioral Reviews. 2012;**36**:1376-1381. DOI: 10.1016/J.NEUBIOREV.2012.02.013

[55] Lee PC, Bordelon Y, Bronstein J, Ritz B. Traumatic brain injury, paraquat exposure, and their relationship to Parkinson disease. Neurology. 2012;**79**:2061-2066. DOI: 10.1212/WNL.0B013E3182749F28

[56] Dams-O'Connor K, Gibbons LE, Bowen JD, McCurry SM, Larson EB, Crane PK. Risk for late-life re-injury, dementia and death among individuals with traumatic brain injury: A population-based study. Journal of Neurology, Neurosurgery, and Psychiatry. 2013;**84**:177-182. DOI: 10.1136/JNNP-2012-303938

[57] Hu W, Tung YC, Zhang Y, Liu F, Iqbal K. Involvement of activation of asparaginyl endopeptidase in tau hyperphosphorylation in repetitive mild traumatic brain injury. Journal of Alzheimer's Disease. 2018;**64**:709. DOI: 10.3233/JAD-180177

[58] Marklund N, Vedung F, Lubberink M, Tegner Y, Johansson J, Blennow K, et al. Tau aggregation and increased neuroinflammation in athletes after sports-related concussions and in traumatic brain injury patients - a PET/MR study. NeuroImage: Clinical. 2021;**30**:102665. DOI: 10.1016/J.NICL.2021.102665

[59] Zemlan FP, Rosenberg WS, Luebbe PA, Campbell TA, Dean GE, Weiner NE, et al. Quantification of axonal damage in traumatic brain injury: Affinity purification and characterization of cerebrospinal fluid tau proteins. Journal of Neurochemistry. 1999;**72**:741-750. DOI: 10.1046/J.1471-4159.1999.0720741.X

[60] Zemlan FP, Jauch EC, Mulchahey JJ, Gabbita SP, Rosenberg WS, Speciale SG, et al. C-tau biomarker of neuronal damage in severe brain injured patients: Association with elevated intracranial pressure and clinical outcome. Brain Research. 2002;**947**:131-139. DOI: 10.1016/S0006-8993(02)02920-7

[61] Smith DH, Chen XH, Nonaka M, Trojanowski JQ, Lee VMY, Saatman KE, et al. Accumulation of amyloid beta and tau and the formation of neurofilament inclusions following diffuse brain injury in the pig. Journal of Neuropathology and Experimental Neurology. 1999;**58**:982-992. DOI: 10.1097/00005072-199909000-00008

[62] Pandey S, Singh K, Sharma V, Pandey D, Jha RP, Rai SK, et al. A prospective pilot study on serum cleaved tau protein as a neurological marker in severe traumatic brain injury. British Journal of Neurosurgery.

2017;**31**:356-363. DOI: 10.1080/02688697.2017.1297378

[63] Ballard C, Gauthier S, Corbett A, Brayne C, Aarsland D, Jones E. Alzheimer's disease. Lancet (London, England). 2011;**377**:1019-1031. DOI: 10.1016/S0140-6736(10)61349-9

[64] Wang J, Gu BJ, Masters CL, Wang YJ. A systemic view of Alzheimer disease - insights from amyloid-β metabolism beyond the brain. Nature Reviews. Neurology. 2017;**13**:612-623. DOI: 10.1038/nrneurol.2017.111

[65] Liu PP, Xie Y, Meng XY, Kang JS. History and progress of hypotheses and clinical trials for Alzheimer's disease. Signal Transduction and Targeted Therapy. 2019;**4**(1):1-22. DOI: 10.1038/s41392-019-0063-8

[66] Scheltens P, Blennow K, Breteler MMB, de Strooper B, Frisoni GB, Salloway S, et al. Alzheimer's disease. Lancet (London, England). 2016;**388**:505-517. DOI: 10.1016/S0140-6736(15)01124-1

[67] Xu J, Rasmussen IA, Lagopoulos J, Haberg A. Diffuse axonal injury in severe traumatic brain injury visualized using high-resolution diffusion tensor imaging. Journal of Neurotrauma. 2007;**24**:753-765. DOI: 10.1089/NEU.2006.0208

[68] Deber CM, Reynolds SJ. Central nervous system myelin: Structure, function, and pathology. Clinical Biochemistry. 1991;**24**:113-134. DOI: 10.1016/0009-9120(91)90421-A

[69] Ming CL, Akle V, Zheng W, Kitlen J, O'Steen B, Larner SF, et al. Extensive degradation of myelin basic protein isoforms by calpain following traumatic brain injury. Journal of Neurochemistry. 2006;**98**:700-712. DOI: 10.1111/J.1471-4159.2006.03882.X

[70] Ottens AK, Golden EC, Bustamante L, Hayes RL, Denslow ND, Wang KKW. Proteolysis of multiple myelin basic protein isoforms after neurotrauma: Characterization by mass spectrometry. Journal of Neurochemistry. 2008;**104**:1404-1414. DOI: 10.1111/J.1471-4159.2007.05086.X

[71] Thomas DGT, Palfreyman JW, Ratcliffe JG. Serum-myelin-basic-protein assay in diagnosis and prognosis of patients with head injury. Lancet (London, England). 1978;**1**:113-115. DOI: 10.1016/S0140-6736(78)90415-4

[72] Berger RP, Adelson PD, Pierce MC, Dulani T, Cassidy LD, Kochanek PM. Serum neuron-specific enolase, S100B, and myelin basic protein concentrations after inflicted and noninflicted traumatic brain injury in children. Journal of Neurosurgery. 2005;**103**:61-68. DOI: 10.3171/PED.2005.103.1.0061

[73] Beers SR, Berger RP, Adelson PD. Neurocognitive outcome and serum biomarkers in inflicted versus non-inflicted traumatic brain injury in young children. Journal of Neurotrauma. 2007;**24**:97-105. DOI: 10.1089/NEU.2006.0055

[74] Giacoppo S, Bramanti P, Barresi M, Celi D, Cuzzola VF, Palella E, et al. Predictive biomarkers of recovery in traumatic brain injury. Neurocritical Care. 2012;**16**:470-477. DOI: 10.1007/S12028-012-9707-Z

[75] Yamazaki Y, Ohtaka H, Morii S, Kitahara T, Ohwada T, Yada K. Diagnostic significance of serum neuron-specific enolase and myelin basic protein assay in patients with acute head injury. Surgical Neurology. 1995;**43**:381-383. DOI: 10.1007/978-4-431-68231-8_86

[76] Mehta T, Fayyaz M, Giler GE, Kaur H, Raikwar SP, Kempuraj D,

et al. Current trends in biomarkers for traumatic brain injury. Open Access Journal of Neurology & Neurosurgery. 2020;**12**:86

[77] Wallimann T, Hemmer W. Creatine kinase in non-muscle tissues and cells. Molecular and Cellular Biochemistry. 1994;**133-134**:193-220. DOI: 10.1007/BF01267955

[78] Rabow L, Hedman G. CKBB-isoenzymes as a sign of cerebral injury. Acta Neurochirurgica. Supplementum (Wien). 1979;**28**:108-112. DOI: 10.1007/978-3-7091-4088-8_24

[79] Kaste M, Hernesniemi J, Somer H, Hillbom M, Konttinen A. Creatine kinase isoenzymes in acute brain injury. Journal of Neurosurgery. 1981;**55**:511-515. DOI: 10.3171/JNS.1981.55.4.0511

[80] Rabow L, DeSalles AAF, Becker DP, Yang M, Kontos HA, Ward JD, et al. CSF brain creatine kinase levels and lactic acidosis in severe head injury. Journal of Neurosurgery. 1986;**65**:625-629. DOI: 10.3171/JNS.1986.65.5.0625

[81] Skogseid IM, Nordby HK, Urdal P, Paus E, Lilleaas F. Increased serum creatine kinase BB and neuron specific enolase following head injury indicates brain damage. Acta Neurochirurgica. 1992;**115**:106-111. DOI: 10.1007/BF01406367

[82] Mussack T, Kirchhoff C, Buhmann S, Biberthaler P, Ladurner R, Gippner-Steppert C, et al. Significance of Elecsys S100 immunoassay for real-time assessment of traumatic brain damage in multiple trauma patients. Clinical Chemistry and Laboratory Medicine. 2006;**44**:1140-1145. DOI: 10.1515/CCLM.2006.190

[83] Stopfkuchen H, Schranz D, Salzmann G, Jüngst BK, Wiss M, Schwarz M. The diagnostic value of CK-MB isoenzyme determinations in children with head injury and polytrauma. Monatsschrift für Kinderheilkunde. 1984;**132**:594-599

[84] Kärkelä J, Bock E, Kaukinen S. CSF and serum brain-specific creatine kinase isoenzyme (CK-BB), neuron-specific enolase (NSE) and neural cell adhesion molecule (NCAM) as prognostic markers for hypoxic brain injury after cardiac arrest in man. Journal of the Neurological Sciences. 1993;**116**:100-109. DOI: 10.1016/0022-510X(93)90095-G

[85] Morris MC, Bercz A, Niziolek GM, Kassam F, Veile R, Friend LA, et al. UCH-L1 is a poor serum biomarker of murine traumatic brain injury after polytrauma. The Journal of Surgical Research. 2019;**244**:63-68. DOI: 10.1016/J.JSS.2019.06.023

[86] Berger RP, Pierce MC, Wisniewski SR, Adelson PD, Clark RSB, Ruppel RA, et al. Neuron-specific enolase and S100B in cerebrospinal fluid after severe traumatic brain injury in infants and children. Pediatrics. 2002;**109**:E31. DOI: 10.1542/PEDS.109.2.E31

[87] Liu M, Zhang C, Liu W, Luo P, Zhang L, Wang Y, et al. A novel rat model of blast-induced traumatic brain injury simulating different damage degree: Implications for morphological, neurological, and biomarker changes. Frontiers in Cellular Neuroscience. 2015;**9**:168. DOI: 10.3389/FNCEL.2015.00168

[88] Verfaillie CJ, Delanghe JR. Hemolysis correction factor in the measurement of serum neuron-specific enolase. Clinical Chemistry and Laboratory Medicine. 2010;**48**:891-892. DOI: 10.1515/CCLM.2010.159

[89] Pfeifer R, Börner A, Krack A, Sigusch HH, Surber R, Figulla HR. Outcome after cardiac arrest: Predictive values and limitations of the neuroproteins neuron-specific enolase and protein S-100 and the Glasgow coma scale. Resuscitation. 2005;**65**:49-55. DOI: 10.1016/J.RESUSCITATION.2004.10.011

[90] Pelinka LE, Jafarmadar M, Redl H, Bahrami S. Neuron-specific-enolase is increased in plasma after hemorrhagic shock and after bilateral femur fracture without traumatic brain injury in the rat. Shock. 2004;**22**:88-91. DOI: 10.1097/01.SHK.0000130157.34382.3F

[91] Wolf H, Krall C, Pajenda G, Leitgeb J, Bukaty AJ, Hajdu S, et al. Alterations of the biomarker S-100B and NSE in patients with acute vertebral spine fractures. The Spine Journal. 2014;**14**:2918-2922. DOI: 10.1016/j.spinee.2014.04.027

[92] Kok WF, Koerts J, Tucha O, Scheeren TWL, Absalom AR. Neuronal damage biomarkers in the identification of patients at risk of long-term postoperative cognitive dysfunction after cardiac surgery. Anaesthesia. 2017;**72**:359-369. DOI: 10.1111/ANAE.13712

[93] Yuan X, Wang J, Wang D, Yang S, Yu N, Guo F. NSE, S100B and MMP9 expression following reperfusion after carotid artery stenting. Current Neurovascular Research. 2019;**16**:129-134. DOI: 10.2174/1567202616666190321123515

[94] Zhang X, Ma S, Chen Y, Yin Y, Bai W, Tan J, et al. The isocitrate dehydrogenase 1 is a potential prognostic indicator for non-small cell lung cancer patients. The International Journal of Biological Markers. 2021;**36**:27-35. DOI: 10.1177/17246008211052571

[95] Missler U, Orlowski N, Nötzold A, Dibbelt L, Steinmeier E, Wiesmann M. Early elevation of S-100B protein in blood after cardiac surgery is not a predictor of ischemic cerebral injury. Clinica Chimica Acta. 2002;**321**:29-33. DOI: 10.1016/S0009-8981(02)00061-X

[96] Okonkwo DO, Yue JK, Puccio AM, Panczykowski DM, Inoue T, McMahon PJ, et al. GFAP-BDP as an acute diagnostic marker in traumatic brain injury: Results from the prospective transforming research and clinical knowledge in traumatic brain injury study. Journal of Neurotrauma. 2013;**30**:1490-1497. DOI: 10.1089/NEU.2013.2883

[97] Yang Z, Wang KKW. Glial fibrillary acidic protein: From intermediate filament assembly and gliosis to neurobiomarker. Trends in Neurosciences. 2015;**38**:364-374. DOI: 10.1016/J.TINS.2015.04.003

[98] Adrian H, Mårten K, Salla N, Lasse V. Biomarkers of traumatic brain injury: Temporal changes in body fluids. ENeuro. 2016;**3**:ENEURO.0294-16.2016. DOI: 10.1523/ENEURO.0294-16.2016

[99] Nylén K, Öst M, Csajbok LZ, Nilsson I, Blennow K, Nellgård B, et al. Increased serum-GFAP in patients with severe traumatic brain injury is related to outcome. Journal of the Neurological Sciences. 2006;**240**:85-91. DOI: 10.1016/J.JNS.2005.09.007

[100] Diaz-Arrastia R, Wang KKW, Papa L, Sorani MD, Yue JK, Puccio AM, et al. Acute biomarkers of traumatic brain injury: Relationship between plasma levels of ubiquitin C-terminal hydrolase-L1 and glial fibrillary acidic protein. Journal of Neurotrauma. 2014;**31**:19-25. DOI: 10.1089/NEU.2013.3040

[101] Hainfellner JA, Voigtländer T, Ströbel T, Mazal PR, Maddalena AS, Aguzzi A, et al. Fibroblasts can express glial fibrillary acidic protein (GFAP) in vivo. Journal of Neuropathology and Experimental Neurology. 2001;**60**:449-461. DOI: 10.1093/JNEN/60.5.449

[102] Posti JP, Hossain I, Takala RSK, Liedes H, Newcombe V, Outtrim J, et al. Glial fibrillary acidic protein and ubiquitin C-terminal hydrolase-L1 are not specific biomarkers for mild CT-negative traumatic brain injury. Journal of Neurotrauma. 2017;**34**:1427-1438. DOI: 10.1089/NEU.2016.4442

[103] Shemilt M, Boutin A, Lauzier F, Zarychanski R, Moore L, McIntyre LA, et al. Prognostic value of glial fibrillary acidic protein in patients with moderate and severe traumatic brain injury: A systematic review and meta-analysis. Critical Care Medicine. 2019;**47**:e522-e529. DOI: 10.1097/CCM.0000000000003728

[104] Lei J, Gao G, Feng J, Jin Y, Wang C, Mao Q, et al. Glial fibrillary acidic protein as a biomarker in severe traumatic brain injury patients: A prospective cohort study. Critical Care. 2015;**19**:1-12. DOI: 10.1186/S13054-015-1081-8/TABLES/3

[105] Fraser DD, Close TE, Rose KL, Ward R, Mehl M, Farrell C, et al. Severe traumatic brain injury in children elevates glial fibrillary acidic protein in cerebrospinal fluid and serum. Pediatric Critical Care Medicine. 2011;**12**:319-324. DOI: 10.1097/PCC.0B013E3181E8B32D

[106] Olsson B, Zetterberg H, Hampel H, Blennow K. Biomarker-based dissection of neurodegenerative diseases. Progress in Neurobiology. 2011;**95**:520-534. DOI: 10.1016/J.PNEUROBIO.2011.04.006

[107] Persson L, Hårdemark HG, Gustafsson J, Rundström G, Mendel-Hartvig I, Esscher T, et al. S-100 protein and neuron-specific enolase in cerebrospinal fluid and serum: Markers of cell damage in human central nervous system. Stroke. 1987;**18**:911-918. DOI: 10.1161/01.STR.18.5.911

[108] Xiong H, Liang WL, Wu XR. Pathophysiological alterations in cultured astrocytes exposed to hypoxia/reoxygenation. Sheng Li Ke Xue Jin Zhan. 2000;**31**:217-221

[109] Donato R, Sorci G, Riuzzi F, Arcuri C, Bianchi R, Brozzi F, et al. S100B's double life: Intracellular regulator and extracellular signal. Biochimica et Biophysica Acta. 2009;**1793**:1008-1022. DOI: 10.1016/J.BBAMCR.2008.11.009

[110] Michetti F, D'Ambrosi N, Toesca A, Puglisi MA, Serrano A, Marchese E, et al. The S100B story: From biomarker to active factor in neural injury. Journal of Neurochemistry. 2019;**148**:168-187. DOI: 10.1111/JNC.14574

[111] Einav S, Shoshan Y, Ovadia H, Matot I, Hersch M, Itshayek E. Early postoperative serum S100β levels predict ongoing brain damage after meningioma surgery: A prospective observational study. Critical Care. 2006;**10**:1-10. DOI: 10.1186/CC5058/FIGURES/4

[112] Anczykowski G, Kaczmarek J, Jankowski R, Guzniczak P. The reference level of serum S-100B protein for poor prognosis in patients with intracranial extracerebral hematoma. EJIFCC. 2011;**22**:66

[113] Grevfors N, Lindblad C, Nelson DW, Svensson M, Thelin EP, Rubenson WR. Delayed neurosurgical intervention in traumatic brain injury patients referred from primary hospitals is not associated with an unfavorable outcome. Frontiers in

Neurology. 2021;**11**:1799. DOI: 10.3389/FNEUR.2020.610192

[114] Chen YH, Cheng ZY, Shao LH, Shentu HS, Fu B. Macrophage migration inhibitory factor as a serum prognostic marker in patients with aneurysmal subarachnoid hemorrhage. Clinica Chimica Acta. 2017;**473**:60-64. DOI: 10.1016/J.CCA.2017.08.018

[115] Jönsson H, Johnsson P, Höglund P, Alling C, Blomquist S. Elimination of S100B and renal function after cardiac surgery. Journal of Cardiothoracic and Vascular Anesthesia. 2000;**14**:698-701. DOI: 10.1053/JCAN.2000.18444

[116] Papa L, Silvestri S, Brophy GM, Giordano P, Falk JL, Braga CF, et al. GFAP out-performs S100β in detecting traumatic intracranial lesions on computed tomography in trauma patients with mild traumatic brain injury and those with extracranial lesions. Journal of Neurotrauma. 2014;**31**:1815-1822. DOI: 10.1089/NEU.2013.3245

[117] Metting Z, Wilczak N, Rodiger LA, Schaaf JM, Van Der Naalt J. GFAP and S100B in the acute phase of mild traumatic brain injury. Neurology. 2012;**78**:1428-1433. DOI: 10.1212/WNL.0B013E318253D5C7

[118] Barbosa RR, Jawa R, Watters JM, Knight JC, Kerwin AJ, Winston ES, et al. Evaluation and management of mild traumatic brain injury: An eastern Association for the Surgery of trauma practice management guideline. Journal of Trauma and Acute Care Surgery. 2012;**73**:S307-S314. DOI: 10.1097/TA.0B013E3182701885

[119] Zongo D, Ribéreau-Gayon R, Masson F, Laborey M, Contrand B, Salmi LR, et al. S100-B protein as a screening tool for the early assessment of minor head injury. Annals of Emergency Medicine. 2012;**59**:209-218. DOI: 10.1016/J.ANNEMERGMED.2011.07.027

[120] Rothoerl RD, Woertgen C, Holzschuh M, Metz C, Brawanski A. S-100 serum levels after minor and major head injury. The Journal of Trauma. 1998;**45**:765-767. DOI: 10.1097/00005373-199810000-00025

[121] Herrmann M, Curio N, Jost S, Wunderlich MT, Synowitz H, Wallesch CW. Protein S-100B and neuron specific enolase as early neurobiochemical markers of the severity of traumatic brain injury. Restorative Neurology and Neuroscience. 1999;**14**:109-114

[122] Biberthaler P, Musaelyan K, Krieg S, Meyer B, Stimmer H, Zapf J, et al. Evaluation of acute glial fibrillary acidic protein and ubiquitin C-terminal hydrolase-L1 plasma levels in traumatic brain injury patients with and without intracranial lesions. Neurotrauma Reports. 2021;**2**:617. DOI: 10.1089/NEUR.2021.0048

[123] Da Rocha AB, Schneider RF, De Freitas GR, André C, Grivicich I, Zanoni C, et al. Role of serum S100B as a predictive marker of fatal outcome following isolated severe head injury or multitrauma in males. Clinical Chemistry and Laboratory Medicine. 2006;**44**:1234-1242. DOI: 10.1515/CCLM.2006.218

[124] Rodríguez-Rodríguez A, Egea-Guerrero JJ, León-Justel A, Gordillo-Escobar E, Revuelto-Rey J, Vilches-Arenas Á, et al. Role of S100B protein in urine and serum as an early predictor of mortality after severe traumatic brain injury in adults. Clinica Chimica Acta. 2012;**414**:228-233. DOI: 10.1016/J.CCA.2012.09.025

[125] Gradisek P, Osredkar J, Korsic M, Kremzar B. Multiple indicators model of

long-term mortality in traumatic brain injury. Brain Injury. 2012;**26**:1472-1481. DOI: 10.3109/02699052.2012.694567

[126] Raheja A, Sinha S, Samson N, Bhoi S, Subramanian A, Sharma P, et al. Serum biomarkers as predictors of long-term outcome in severe traumatic brain injury: Analysis from a randomized placebo-controlled phase II clinical trial. Journal of Neurosurgery. 2016;**125**:631-641. DOI: 10.3171/2015.6.JNS15674

[127] Thelin EP, Frostell A, Mulder J, Mitsios N, Damberg P, Aski SN, et al. Lesion size is exacerbated in hypoxic rats whereas hypoxia-inducible factor-1 alpha and vascular endothelial growth factor increase in injured normoxic rats: A prospective cohort study of secondary hypoxia in focal traumatic brain injury. Frontiers in Neurology. 2016;7:23. DOI: 10.3389/FNEUR.2016.00023

[128] Rainey T, Lesko M, Sacho R, Lecky F, Childs C. Predicting outcome after severe traumatic brain injury using the serum S100B biomarker: Results using a single (24h) time-point. Resuscitation. 2009;**80**:341-345. DOI: 10.1016/J.RESUSCITATION.2008.11.021

[129] Egea-Guerrero JJ, Murillo-Cabezas F, Gordillo-EscobarE, Rodríguez-RodríguezA, Enamorado-Enamorado J, Revuelto-Rey J, et al. S100B protein may detect brain death development after severe traumatic brain injury. Journal of Neurotrauma. 2013;**30**:1762. DOI: 10.1089/NEU.2012.2606

[130] Kellermann I, Kleindienst A, Hore N, Buchfelder M, Brandner S. Early CSF and serum S100B concentrations for outcome prediction in traumatic brain injury and subarachnoid hemorrhage. Clinical Neurology and Neurosurgery. 2016;**145**:79-83. DOI: 10.1016/J.CLINEURO.2016.04.005

[131] Thelin EP, Johannesson L, Nelson D, Bellander BM. S100B is an important outcome predictor in traumatic brain injury. Journal of Neurotrauma. 2013;**30**:519-528. DOI: 10.1089/NEU.2012.2553

[132] Park SH, Hwang SK. Prognostic value of serum levels of S100 calcium-binding protein B, neuron-specific enolase, and interleukin-6 in pediatric patients with traumatic brain injury. World Neurosurgery. 2018;**118**:e534-e542. DOI: 10.1016/J.WNEU.2018.06.234

[133] Yin W, Weng S, Lai S, Nie H. GCS score combined with CT score and serum S100B protein level can evaluate severity and early prognosis of acute traumatic brain injury. Nan Fang Yi Ke Da Xue Xue Bao. 2021;**41**:543-548. DOI: 10.12122/J.ISSN.1673-4254.2021.04.09

[134] Korfias S, Stranjalis G, Boviatsis E, Psachoulia C, Jullien G, Gregson B, et al. Serum S-100B protein monitoring in patients with severe traumatic brain injury. Intensive Care Medicine. 2007;**33**:255-260. DOI: 10.1007/S00134-006-0463-4

[135] Taheri A, Emami M, Asadipour E, Kasirzadeh S, Rouini MR, Najafi A, et al. A randomized controlled trial on the efficacy, safety, and pharmacokinetics of metformin in severe traumatic brain injury. Journal of Neurology. 2019;**266**:1988-1997. DOI: 10.1007/S00415-019-09366-1

[136] Thelin EP, Nelson DW, Bellander BM. Secondary peaks of S100B in serum relate to subsequent radiological pathology in traumatic brain injury. Neurocritical Care. 2014;**20**:217-229. DOI: 10.1007/S12028-013-9916-0

[137] Di Battista AP, Buonora JE, Rhind SG, Hutchison MG, Baker AJ,

Rizoli SB, et al. Blood biomarkers in moderate-to-severe traumatic brain injury: Potential utility of a multi-marker approach in characterizing outcome. Frontiers in Neurology. 2015;**6**:110. DOI: 10.3389/FNEUR.2015.00110

[138] Lee JY, Lee CY, Kim HR, Lee CH, Kim HW, Kim JH. A role of serum-based neuronal and glial markers as potential predictors for distinguishing severity and related outcomes in traumatic brain injury. Journal of Korean Neurosurgical Association. 2015;**58**:93-100. DOI: 10.3340/JKNS.2015.58.2.93

[139] Thelin EP, Nelson DW, Bellander BM. A review of the clinical utility of serum S100B protein levels in the assessment of traumatic brain injury. Acta Neurochirurgica. 2017;**159**:209-225. DOI: 10.1007/S00701-016-3046-3

[140] Bloomfield SM, McKinney J, Smith L, Brisman J. Reliability of S100B in predicting severity of central nervous system injury. Neurocritical Care. 2007;**6**:121-138. DOI: 10.1007/S12028-007-0008-X

[141] Pham N, Fazio V, Cucullo L, Teng Q, Biberthaler P, Bazarian JJ, et al. Extracranial sources of S100B do not affect serum levels. PLoS One. 2010;**5**:e12691. DOI: 10.1371/JOURNAL.PONE.0012691

[142] Piazza O, Storti MP, Cotena S, Stoppa F, Perrotta D, Esposito G, et al. S100B is not a reliable prognostic index in paediatric TBI. Pediatric Neurosurgery. 2007;**43**:258-264. DOI: 10.1159/000103304

[143] Papa L, Edwards D, Ramia M. Exploring serum biomarkers for mild traumatic brain injury. In: Brain Neurotrauma: Molecular, Neuropsychological, and Rehabilitation Aspects. Boca Raton (FL): CRC Press; 2015. pp. 301-308. DOI: 10.1201/b18126

[144] Blennow K, Zetterberg H. The past and the future of Alzheimer's disease fluid biomarkers. Journal of Alzheimer's Disease. 2018;**62**:1125-1140. DOI: 10.3233/JAD-170773

[145] Li J, Yu C, Sun Y, Li Y. Serum ubiquitin C-terminal hydrolase L1 as a biomarker for traumatic brain injury: A systematic review and meta-analysis. The American Journal of Emergency Medicine. 2015;**33**:1191-1196. DOI: 10.1016/J.AJEM.2015.05.023

[146] Janigro D, Bailey DM, Lehmann S, Badaut J, O'Flynn R, Hirtz C, et al. Peripheral blood and salivary biomarkers of blood-brain barrier permeability and neuronal damage: Clinical and applied concepts. Frontiers in Neurology. 2021;**11**:577312. DOI: 10.3389/FNEUR.2020.577312

[147] Rogatzki MJ, Morgan JE, Baker JS, Knox A, Serrador JM. Protein S100B and brain lipid-binding protein concentrations in the serum of recently concussed rugby players. Journal of Neurotrauma. 2021;**38**:2247-2254. DOI: 10.1089/NEU.2021.0004

[148] Larsen CN, Price JS, Wilkinson KD. Substrate binding and catalysis by ubiquitin C-terminal hydrolases: Identification of two active site residues. Biochemistry. 1996;**35**: 6735-6744. DOI: 10.1021/BI960099F

[149] Kobeissy FH, Ottens AK, Zhang Z, Liu MC, Denslow ND, Dave JR, et al. Novel differential neuroproteomics analysis of traumatic brain injury in rats. Molecular & Cellular Proteomics. 2006;**5**:1887-1898. DOI: 10.1074/MCP.M600157-MCP200

[150] Liu MC, Akinyi L, Scharf D, Mo J, Larner SF, Muller U, et al. Ubiquitin

C-terminal hydrolase-L1 as a biomarker for ischemic and traumatic brain injury in rats. The European Journal of Neuroscience. 2010;**31**:722-732. DOI: 10.1111/J.1460-9568.2010.07097.X

[151] Papa L, Brophy GM, Welch RD, Lewis LM, Braga CF, Tan CN, et al. Time course and diagnostic accuracy of glial and neuronal blood biomarkers GFAP and UCH-L1 in a large cohort of trauma patients with and without mild traumatic brain injury. JAMA Neurology. 2016;**73**:551-560. DOI: 10.1001/JAMANEUROL.2016.0039

[152] Bazarian JJ, Biberthaler P, Welch RD, Lewis LM, Barzo P, Bogner-Flatz V, et al. Serum GFAP and UCH-L1 for prediction of absence of intracranial injuries on head CT (ALERT-TBI): A multicentre observational study. Lancet Neurology. 2018;**17**:782-789. DOI: 10.1016/S1474-4422(18)30231-X

[153] Richard M, Lagares A, Bondanese V, De La Cruz J, Mejan O, Pavlov V, et al. Study protocol for investigating the performance of an automated blood test measuring GFAP and UCH-L1 in a prospective observational cohort of patients with mild traumatic brain injury: European BRAINI study. BMJ Open. 2021;**11**:e043635. DOI: 10.1136/BMJOPEN-2020-043635

[154] Papa L, Akinyi L, Liu MC, Pineda JA, Tepas JJ, Oli MW, et al. Ubiquitin C-terminal hydrolase is a novel biomarker in humans for severe traumatic brain injury. Critical Care Medicine. 2010;**38**:138-144. DOI: 10.1097/CCM.0B013E3181B788AB

[155] Mondello S, Linnet A, Buki A, Robicsek S, Gabrielli A, Tepas J, et al. Clinical utility of serum levels of ubiquitin C-terminal hydrolase as a biomarker for severe traumatic brain injury. Neurosurgery. 2012;**70**:666-675. DOI: 10.1227/neu.0b013e318236a809

[156] Zhang R, Zhang CY, Zhao Q, Li DH. Spectrin: Structure, function and disease. Science China. Life Sciences. 2013;**56**:1076-1085. DOI: 10.1007/S11427-013-4575-0

[157] Wang KKW, Posmantur R, Nath R, McGinnist K, Whitton M, Talanian RV, et al. Simultaneous degradation of alphaII- and betaII-spectrin by caspase 3 (CPP32) in apoptotic cells. The Journal of Biological Chemistry. 1998;**273**:22490-22497. DOI: 10.1074/JBC.273.35.22490

[158] Pike BR, Zhao X, Newcomb JK, Posmantur RM, Wang KKW, Hayes RL. Regional calpain and caspase-3 proteolysis of alpha-spectrin after traumatic brain injury. Neuroreport. 1998;**9**:2437-2442. DOI: 10.1097/00001756-199808030-00002

[159] Pineda JA, Wang KKW, Hayes RL. Biomarkers of proteolytic damage following traumatic brain injury. Brain Pathology. 2004;**14**:202-209. DOI: 10.1111/J.1750-3639.2004.TB00054.X

[160] Farkas O, Polgár B, Szekeres-Barthó J, Dóczi T, Povlishock JT, Büki A. Spectrin breakdown products in the cerebrospinal fluid in severe head injury--preliminary observations. Acta Neurochirurgica. 2005;**147**:855-860. DOI: 10.1007/S00701-005-0559-6

[161] Svetlov SI, Larner SF, Kirk DR, Atkinson J, Hayes RL, Wang KKW. Biomarkers of blast-induced neurotrauma: Profiling molecular and cellular mechanisms of blast brain injury. Journal of Neurotrauma. 2009;**26**:913. DOI: 10.1089/NEU.2008.0609

[162] Li J, Li XY, Feng DF, Pan DC. Biomarkers associated with diffuse traumatic axonal injury: Exploring pathogenesis, early diagnosis, and

prognosis. The Journal of Trauma. 2010;**69**:1610-1618. DOI: 10.1097/TA.0B013E3181F5A9ED

[163] Zetterberg H. Neurofilament light: A dynamic cross-disease fluid biomarker for neurodegeneration. Neuron. 2016;**91**:1-3. DOI: 10.1016/J.NEURON.2016.06.030

[164] Gaetani L, Blennow K, Calabresi P, Di Filippo M, Parnetti L, Zetterberg H. Neurofilament light chain as a biomarker in neurological disorders. Journal of Neurology, Neurosurgery, and Psychiatry. 2019;**90**:870-881. DOI: 10.1136/JNNP-2018-320106

[165] Van Geel WJA, Rosengren LE, Verbeek MM. An enzyme immunoassay to quantify neurofilament light chain in cerebrospinal fluid. Journal of Immunological Methods. 2005;**296**:179-185. DOI: 10.1016/J.JIM.2004.11.015

[166] Laverse E, Guo T, Zimmerman K, Foiani MS, Velani B, Morrow P, et al. Plasma glial fibrillary acidic protein and neurofilament light chain, but not tau, are biomarkers of sports-related mild traumatic brain injury. Brain Communications. 2020;**2**:fcaa137. DOI: 10.1093/BRAINCOMMS/FCAA137

[167] Shahim P, Politis A, van der Merwe A, Moore B, Ekanayake V, Lippa SM, et al. Time course and diagnostic utility of NfL, tau, GFAP, and UCH-L1 in subacute and chronic TBI. Neurology. 2020;**95**:e623-e636. DOI: 10.1212/WNL.0000000000009985

[168] Shahim P, Politis A, van der Merwe A, Moore B, Chou YY, Pham DL, et al. Neurofilament light as a biomarker in traumatic brain injury. Neurology. 2020;**95**:e610-e622. DOI: 10.1212/WNL.0000000000009983

[169] Anderson KJ, Scheff SW, Miller KM, Roberts KN, Gilmer LK, Yang C, et al. The phosphorylated axonal form of the neurofilament subunit NF-H (pNF-H) as a blood biomarker of traumatic brain injury. Journal of Neurotrauma. 2008;**25**:1079-1085. DOI: 10.1089/NEU.2007.0488